BETTER!

11 SIMPLE HABITS TO IMPROVE YOUR LIFE

DR. JASON PIKEN
D.C., C.N.S.

"I've been a patient of Dr. Piken since 2005. I couldn't be happier with my experience and am grateful for Dr. Piken's wisdom, open-mindedness, and dedication to empowering patients and giving us the tools to heal, whether that's an adjustment, nutritional advice, or laser therapy. . . . Dr. Piken has been an invaluable friend, guide, and partner in health."

—Lauren U.

"I didn't think about looking for a chiropractor when I was searching for the answers to why my body didn't want to keep up with me. Dr Piken was recommended to me by another chiropractor and it was the best ...Morel didn't think about looking for a chiropractor when I was searching for the answers to why my body didn't want to keep up with me. Dr. Piken has an amazing understanding of the human body and the person within. For years I've been fighting for my health. I've tried everything and even if some of it worked, it was only a question of time until my body started attacking itself again. His therapy and overall guidance on my physical and emotional health were the tools I needed to get my life back on track. Dr. Piken is a lifesaver!

—Nina Sjögren-Höe

"Doctor Piken has been my primary health caregiver for nearly twenty years because he is never wrong. He is a true healer and one of my personal heroes."

—Stephen M.

"Dr. Piken has a very wholesome approach—he focuses on chiropractic issues along with diet, posture, habits, and overall body health. . . . Dr. Piken changed my life for the better, and I am so thankful!"

—Nyla I.

"I have known Dr. Piken since 2004. He is always encouraging me to unlock my highest potential; my best self."

—*Nelia Watten*

Dr. Piken is not only a doctor but a teacher. His therapy and overall guidance on my physical as well as my emotional well-being has put me on a clear path to healing and living a healthy life."

—*Paulina Apostolides*

"Accolades are in order for the comprehensive understanding and treatment entailed in Dr. Piken's approach to the human body. The overall impact of his work engendered a perceivable transformation, physically, mentally, and emotionally—and successive visits continue to contribute to and enhance an overall sense of well-being. . . . I look forward to continuing my visits, trusting in the remarkable changes that occur as a result of his insights, intuition, adjustments, [and knowledge and incorporation of] nutrition, laser therapy, kinesiology, exercise, and various psychological contributors in assessing any particular ailment."

—*Helen Stratford*

"Dr. Piken taught me and gave me real strategies to manage stress and digestive issues. He improved my quality of life."

—*Suzanne Ciprut*

Editor: Editorial Project Management, KarenRowe.com

Cover Design: Shake Creative, ShakeTampa.com

Inside Layout: Ljiljana Pavkov

Printed in the United States

ISBN: 978-0-9983885-0-2 (international Trade paper edition)

ISBN: 978-0-9983885-1-9 (eBook)

This book is not intended as a substitute for the medical advice of physicians. The reader should regularly consult a physician in matters relating to his/her health and particularly with respect to any symptoms that may require diagnosis or medical attention. This book contains information that is intended to help the readers be better-informed consumers of healthcare. It is presented as general advice on healthcare. Always consult your doctor for individual needs.

BETTER!

To my wife, Stacey.
No one else on earth knows me the way you do.
Thank you for supporting me, challenging me,
loving me and being my best friend.

To my daughters, Ryan and Avery.
One of the many reasons I wrote this book is so
that you could one day have a tool when you
decide that all of those pain in the butt lessons
your dad annoyed you with made sense and you
want to remember them.

Table of Contents

Acknowledgements

I would like to acknowledge all the people in my life who have allowed me to learn from them, but I would have to write another book to list them all. I have learned something from every person and every experience. Here is a short list of some who stand out:

Mom, Dad, Michael, Nana, and Poppy.

All those who taught me chiropractic and philosophy.

All those who inspired me to learn more applied kinesiology.

All those involved in teaching me nutrition and functional medicine.

The thousands of patients who have required me to be *better*!

My mentors and coaches.

My team at the office.

And finally, to all of you whose audios I have listened to and whose books, blogs, and research I have read, though I have never met you personally, keep it up, fellow educators. You're changing lives!

Introduction

We all have it in us to make our lives better. We have it in us to improve our relationships, our health, and how we feel on a daily basis.

Improving quality of life is not necessarily about reaching a specific target, although sometimes we do work toward a specific target. If you're working toward winning a race, you are working toward a specific goal. But when it comes to how you're living your life every day, the experiences you have, and how you feel year after year in your life, the important thing is this: that you are simply getting better and better all the time. In order to be happy, we must grow and learn. The day we stop growing and wondering and exploring, we begin the process of dying. This book is about growing, learning, and getting better.

I wrote this book because I want you to realize your potential for health, happiness, and abundance. That will mean something different for you than it does for anybody else reading this book. In today's world of reality TV, consumerism, and social media, we are constantly comparing our lives to the lives of others, but not in any real sense. We are only exposed to the picture-perfect moments that people want us to see—not the reality. I want you to realize that if you care more for yourself and your own personal health, you will achieve a level of personal abundance and pleasure far beyond what the distractions promise and far beyond what you could even imagine.

Our bodies carry an innate intelligence and the ability to self-heal. Our job is to take care of our bodies and promote that self-healing process. The condition of our bodies is the sum total of all of our habits. If we change our habits, we change our bodies, and we change our quality of life. I wrote this book to give you my rules for how to do that. I want you to have a superior quality of life.

Lao Tsu, the figurehead behind Taoism and author of the *I Ching*, which predates the Bible, said, "There is nothing new under the sun." That was written thousands of years ago, and all the messages in this book are based upon principles that have stood the test of time. I have read hundreds of books and countless articles, have listened to lectures, and have meditated for many hundreds of hours, and I've never found any magic potion or saying or solution to the world's problems beyond the simple rules and practices I've given you in this book. I know that what I've learned will help you because the principles that are being taught in this book are eternal.

Everything I've written comes from firsthand experience. I grew up not thinking too much about my health or healthy living, until I started to develop symptoms that forced me to start paying attention. I discovered that by truly looking for an understanding of *why* I had the symptoms I had, I could actually fix the problem rather than just treating it with a pill or surgery. I discovered that the place to look was in the habits I was following daily.

The reason I live my life the way I do is not because my parents brought me up this way, and it's not because of my religious beliefs. I definitely live differently than most Americans, so it's not because of what the neighbors might think, either. It's because I have learned *a lot* in my forty-five years, and I have developed certain rules for myself. Over the years, they have served me well.

There are countless people out there not living up to their potential, and I know there is very little holding them back from having a better life. A lot of the books, CDs, and seminars can push people too hard, motivating them but eventually alienating them with rules that are too rigid. This book is about providing information and a guideline for *you* to create your own rules that work for *you*.

We all set habits or rules for the way we live our lives, and sometimes they're in the form of excuses that keep us stuck in a certain lifestyle, ultimately preventing us from truly being happy. I wrote this book to help you move beyond those excuses and actually start implementing new rules that will effectively serve you.

The first chapter of this book is designed to set you up with the tools you need in order to *succeed* at improving your quality of life. The first step to improvement is knowing where you are now. You have to know how you're doing in the areas of life that are important for health and happiness. And you need a tool that is able to measure your progress as you start making changes in your life. So right away, I'll introduce my Personal Report Card, or PRC, and explain how to create yours and fill it out. You'll put down your current grades in the important areas of life so you can see where you are and define your objectives for where you are going.

Next, I'm going to talk about *rules*. What are the rules we play by in our lives? Through this discussion, you'll start to see that everyone's rules are subjective, and we all make up our own rules for how we want to live. Your rules are like your compass; they impact your decisions and your behavior on a daily basis. Through my own experiences, I've learned what works and what doesn't work when it comes to living a healthy, happy life. I wrote this book to share my rules with you. I feel it's my responsibility to do so. Your rules are your rules. You don't need to adopt every single one of mine, but I strongly encourage you to take on the rules that you think will make a difference in your life. Take them and make them your own.

We'll also talk about habits. We have habits for everything we do. Some habits are great for us, and some not so great. Once we decide we want to start playing by new rules, we have to implement new habits to make those rules a reality. I'll take you through some examples of how to implement new habits, so you can be successful at making lasting changes and seeing real progress.

Next, I'll explain how to bring up your grade in each of the areas on your report card. These recommendations all come down to implementing new habits in each area.

My wish for you is that you will begin to take action! Everyone knows that their lives can be better than where they are today. I designed the Personal Report Card to be a simple grading system and an easy tool you can use to improve any and all aspects of your life. I also hope that you want straight As!

I won't fill you up with tons of statistics and research. I have based this book on over two decades of practice, achieving results with thousands of patients. Follow the rules I talk about in this book: eat right, exercise, drink enough clean water, get plenty of sleep and rest so you can heal, have healthy poop, take care of the frame of your body, meditate, and have lots of fun. That's it! Sure, we can put in other good, healthy habits, but these are the majors. If you do these well, you're going to have much fewer problems in life. That's why I'm glad this book made its way into your hands. With your Personal Report Card, your own redefined rules, and new, healthy habits, you'll be well on your way to improving your quality of life!

The Two Whys to Every Health Problem

The goal with your Personal Report Card is to be improving all the time. Ultimately, you want to get to the point where you have straight As and are implementing all the habits of health and great quality of life. However, this won't happen all at once, and it won't happen on its own. You will not keep improving your health and quality of life unless you make the right changes and work at them. To do that, you need to understand the two issues all health problems come from in the first place. When you understand *the two whys to every health problem*, you'll know what actions to implement in your life to keep improving.

Knowing the two whys is a great motivator. This knowledge both inspires you to make the changes needed to keep improving your health and also lets you know if you're on the right track. You see, there are only two factors that have a gigantic impact on your overall health. Therefore, what you should be doing is finding ways to minimize these whys in your life. These two whys are *inflammation* and *stress*. Really, stress *causes* inflammation, but inflammation is such a big deal that we need to address it as a separate issue. So before we jump into the book, I want to talk a little bit about these two whys so you understand them as the basis for the changes that you're going to be making and implementing with your Personal Report Card. Once you understand these two sources of every health problem, you'll be able to make the right improvements.

Inflammation

First, let's talk a bit about *inflammation*. Inflammation is good—we *need* it. Without inflammation, we'd get infections, the infections would overrun our bodies, and we'd die. We also need inflammation to heal cuts and broken bones. However, because of our modern lifestyles—nutritional factors, environmental factors, our habits (and some genetic factors)—many people are living with a chronic mild to moderate hyper-inflammatory state. What this means is that the inflammation in our bodies is out of control, and we need to normalize it.

How do we impact the level of inflammation in our bodies? Inflammation spirals out of control due mostly to our lifestyle and habits: not exercising, allowing ourselves to get too stressed, getting too little sleep, eating chemicals instead of food, not eating the *right* things—putting too many starchy, sugary things in our bodies rather than nutritious, healing foods—and being exposed to chemicals from pesticide residues. But if you take care of your habits in life and instill healthy lifestyle habits, you can avoid this hyper-inflammatory response and ward off many inflammatory conditions.

The major message of this book is to change your lifestyle now, *before* you end up needing medical attention, surgery, or rehabilitation from inflammation. If you've already developed a heightened inflammatory response, making small changes can have a huge positive effect on your body over time. No matter what point you're starting from, you can change your lifestyle and promote a healthy inflammatory response.

Let's take the example of Howard, a patient I was caring for almost two years before he took the steps needed to change his life. Howard had a poor diet, never exercised, and didn't love his job. These were his major inflammatory triggers. Howard already had poor lab tests: high cholesterol, blood sugar and triglyceride issues, and multiple positive inflammatory and autoimmune markers. Howard first came to my office complaining of neck pain. That is the typical symptom that brings people into my office, some type of ache or pain. I am a chiropractor, after all, and that's what most people believe they should come to me for.

If a patient's pain isn't resolving within a few visits, then there usually is a second or third factor perpetuating their symptoms. Howard resisted change, though. Despite me begging and pleading with him to follow the AI paleo diet (described later in the book), take certain supplements, exercise, meditate, and change his job, he chose to simply come in to get adjusted for his neck pain and get relief for a few days at a time. This "dance" went on for almost two years—Howard coming in and complaining of pain, me teaching him *why* his pain kept returning, and him telling me, "Okay, I'll *try* to be better." I consider myself to be a pretty good educator and motivator, but I also understand that until the person I'm teaching is ready to accept the message being delivered, nothing will change.

What was the turnaround for Howard? Howard got his bloodwork evaluated yet again, and the numbers were worse than ever. When I discussed it with him this time, I saw a light switch go on! I wasn't saying anything different than what I had told him every other week for two years, but now it was sinking in. He felt like crap, his habits were crap, and his labs were even crappier than before, and it finally hit him. He basically said to me, "Okay doc, tell me exactly what to do, and I'll do it!" He had his motivator, his *why*. Twelve weeks later, after following the program we discussed for dietary changes and supplements, his lab work was better than it had been in the previous two years. Twelve weeks erased two years of damage.

Howard still isn't living life perfectly. He still needs to meditate, exercise, and, yes, figure out the job thing, but when he finally stops *trying* to do those things and simply improves his other habits, he will reap the same rewards. Meanwhile, after changing only two of his report card grades—diet and supplements—he has lost over thirty pounds and kept it off for a couple years now, giving him a healthy body composition, and he has maintained great results on his blood tests. Oh, and by the way, he barely has any neck pain any longer.

Stress

The second source of every health problem is *stress.* Stress can be broken up into three categories: physical stress (getting punched in the mouth), chemical stress (smoking cigarettes), and emotional stress (trying to meet a 9 a.m. deadline for the big project at work).

Physical stress

Physical stress is easy to understand. Physical stress results from either too little or too much movement. For example, if you exercise too much, carry a heavy backpack, sleep the wrong way, or experience physical trauma like a car accident, trips, or falls, you are experiencing excess *physical* stress. Of course, you want to minimize physical stresses on your body. How you do that is through *habits.* For example, maintaining good posture is a habit the minimizes physical stress on your body. Become conscious of your posture and the way you're carrying yourself, get to a chiropractor to fix and correct your posture, and work on your muscle tone through exercise. The stronger and fitter you are, the better you're going to be able to hold yourself in the right posture, which will minimize physical stress. Read the chapter on exercise to learn how much exercise is too much.

Now, what's key to note here is that you'll never completely *eliminate* physical stress; you'll never get rid of all
of it, and getting rid of it isn't the goal. The goal is simply
to *minimize* it.

Emotional Stress

We are all very familiar with emotional stress. When you
feel exhausted at the end of the day—sometimes that's
from emotional stress. The feeling of taking on too much
and being overwhelmed contributes to emotional stress. For
example, let's say you're working twelve-hour days five to
six days a week, traveling a lot, and averaging six hours of
interrupted sleep per night—meaning you're only sleeping
solidly for about two to three hours at a time. You may think
you can handle this for a short period of time, but after a
while, that stress will affect your emotional state, and it
will build up, even if you're handling it well at the time.
Just because you handle emotional stress well doesn't mean
you shouldn't reduce your exposure. You may even enjoy
a fast-paced lifestyle like this—but, over time, it takes a toll
on your emotional well-being and your health.

I practice in the center of New York City; I believe my
patient base is a bit more work-stressed than most. The high
pace of life in this country is probably experienced by most,
but NYC tends to be a place where the stress from work is
extraordinarily heightened. I don't think I need to list other sources of emotional stress here. Simply think of all the
things you need to get done over the next week of your life,
and there are your emotional stressors.

Not allowing your body to rest and heal as often as
needed can lead to all kinds of health disturbances. You'll
find solutions in this book to enable you to decrease the
amount of emotional stress in your life. For example:

taking a meditation class, adding another hour of sleep per night, leaving work an hour earlier, and making a complete cut-off from work during personal time. You'll learn simple techniques in this book that will decrease your exposure to stress.

Chemical Stress

Chemical stress comes from your body's response to anything you eat, inhale, or rub onto your skin. It can be caused by eating too much or too little food, food allergies, chemicals in our foods, chemicals we inhale because of the area where we live or work, chemicals in the hair or skin products we use. There are thousands of sources of chemical stressors that we are exposed to daily. You can minimize chemical stress on your body by changing your diet and taking supplements that help with healing and recovery. You'll find out more about diet and supplements throughout this book.

What Can You Do About It

For now, the important thing to remember is that stress (in its three forms) and inflammation are the two sources of every health problem. Therefore, minimizing these three types of stress and minimizing inflammation in your body are key to improving your health and your overall quality of life.

The following is the statement I say to patients over and over and over again. It's the statement I use to answer nearly every health-related question that's asked of me. Here's the typical question: "Doc, why do I have _____? I have never had it before.... Doc, I have _____ pain.

Why do you think I have it?" You can phrase the question any way you want; here's the answer!

The reason you have any and all of your symptoms is because you have accumulated either too much physical, chemical, or emotional stress, and your body is reacting.

That stress has either accumulated over decades and you finally are noticing it, *or* there was an occurrence of acute stress like a car accident, a death in the family, a virus, swallowing poison (etc.). The most likely reason is that the life you were living up until your symptom began was not optimal, and your body simply couldn't handle it any longer. How does your body communicate with you? It gives you a symptom. Pain, itching, swelling, anxiety, bloating, cramps, headaches, constipation, you name it. I've got the answer. Go back and read the underlined statement over and over again until you get it! The single best way to treat your symptoms is to *not* treat your symptoms but instead address the physical, chemical, and emotional stress that has accumulated over your lifetime. As a side note, I do hope you realize that if you're bleeding after a car accident, or you suddenly have the worst pain you've ever felt in your life, it may be a good time to go to the emergency room and get the crisis resolved before you change your habits.

The next section will set you up to start making changes that will help you be more adaptable to the stresses of life—and to keep up with those changes! Then we'll discuss how to make changes in each area of your life that will help you minimize stress and inflammation. While I won't bring up stress and inflammation in every section of this book, the recommendations I am giving you come back to minimizing these two things. That's what the tools in this book are all about.

As you continue reading, remember these two whys of every health problem—know that they are the impetus for every new habit you instill—and take comfort in knowing you are doing the right thing to move away from them and into better health and a better quality of life!

PART I
Getting Started

Chapter 1

What Will You Get Out of Reading this Book?

The goal of this book is to give you the tools to live a healthy life. I want you to create rules that will serve as a compass for you to uncover your greatest potential.

The best way to feel great is to live a healthy lifestyle, and I want you to experience the same fulfillment I have achieved through living a healthy lifestyle.

Taking another point of view, I can understand that a person who skydives, skateboards, parties six nights a week, has multiple sexual partners, and feels very little responsibility or stress may think that *I'm* the one who is missing out. Whatever path you choose, most will agree that there is a happiness factor related to adopting a healthy lifestyle. You feel good when you're taking care of yourself, and you'll feel good when you're following the rules you set for yourself.

While establishing rules is crucial, the most important thing is to make sure your rules are the right fit for *you*. I know another chiropractor who eats *only* organic, and every morsel of food needs to be the best quality. Is that right or wrong? Well, from a health point of view, it can't be wrong, but from a lifestyle point of view for *me*—that would make me miserable. So do I eat *only* organic? *No!* But I do buy as much as will make me happy. What's your threshold? It is probably based on a few factors such as your level of education about healthy living, your financial situation, and the friends or family members you choose to surround yourself with.

If you really want to be healthy and feel great, and the ideas in this book strike a chord with you, then my suggestion would be to find more people who share your views about healthy living. It's much easier to follow your chosen rules when everyone around you is following them too.

Rules don't have to be hard to adopt or follow, unless you are completely changing something you have always done and attempting to do it with no moral support. If too many rules make you miserable, then don't follow all of them. Instead, start with a few changes and develop consistency in implementing new habits. Either way, you're following your rules.

For example, if your rule is, *I'm not going to give up ice cream even though it upsets my stomach*, then go ahead and follow that rule—just make sure you're truly happy with following it. Also, remember that there is this amazing option we have as humans (especially as Americans), and that is the right to *change our minds*. So make your own rules, and make sure those rules make you happy!

This book will serve as a guide for you to do exactly that. It will set you up to create new, healthy habits, give you a grading system so you can track your progress, and, ultimately, give you access to creating a better quality of life for yourself. I'm giving you a condensed version of what I've learned over many years. I know the principles taught here will help you!

Let's get started!

Chapter 2

How to Use this Book

Here are my recommendations for how to get the most out of reading this book. First of all, it's not enough to simply read this book. That will give you *insights*, but it won't give you the *progress* you're looking for. While I go into detail about several areas of life throughout the book, it's not enough to simply know *how* to improve your grade in any given area—the magic is in *how you are keeping track of your progress in each of the areas*. Do the work as it comes up in the book. Don't skip ahead before you finish each section. For example, when you finish reading the section about grading guidelines, go create your own grading guidelines. Make sure you've created your report card and your grading system so you have something to work with.

Secondly, you will only progress if you create a grading system for your report card that pushes you to stretch. I would strongly suggest that you push yourself to grow to be better than where you are now. Don't just do what's already comfortable for you. When setting up your grading guidelines, don't make an A represent where you are now on your good days. Make your A your ideal goal. Stretch yourself.

In terms of setting goals for yourself, go with what makes sense for you. Ask yourself, "How much better do I want to get?" Do you want to do an Ironman Triathlon, or do you just want to be able to cut your toenails without stress? This question will govern your goals and therefore your grading system.

Right now, I have simple goals in life. I want to maintain the lifestyle I currently have. But that's because, years ago, my goals were to get where I am now, and I worked hard to get here. I'm living proof that you can set goals for yourself and actually reach them. But it takes consistent effort, the right tools, and commitment to keep at it. That's why we're doing this work together! Now, my goals are about being healthy well into my future. I want to cut my own toenails when I'm ninety-six because, as nice as it will be to have people around me in case I need them, I genuinely want to be able to care for myself. I want to be able to play with my great-grandchildren, and I want to still be playing golf into my nineties. Most importantly, I want an amazing relationship with my family forever! Set achievable goals for yourself that inspire you and push you to grow.

Throughout this book, I give you my rules for improving your quality of life. I recommend that you create your rules as you go—write down the rules that speak to you most. Put your rules somewhere visible so you see them every day. Rules are only helpful if they're followed. Changing your life is simple, but it often isn't easy. It is easy, however, to fall back into old habits, so keep your rules somewhere you can see them and be reminded of them daily.

A good guideline for your report card is to fill it out quarterly at first until your Health Point Average—or HPA, instead of an academic GPA—is at or close to straight As. If you are in a good place and aren't focused on making big changes in your life, then fill it out once per year at the minimum—think about it as a new year's tool. If you know you need to make changes in your life that you want to measure more often, think about doing it at every solstice: summer, fall, winter, and spring. Whenever the seasons change, think of giving yourself a new report card to evaluate your plan for the next three months.

And last but not least, have fun! A huge part of living a great life is enjoying what you're doing. Start now! This is meant to be a fun journey. Just think, you're already on your way to getting better in every area of your life!

PART II
Dr. Piken's Personal Report Card

Chapter 3

Create Your Personal Report Card

In this section, I'm going to take you through the most valuable tool I can give you for improving your quality of life: your Personal Report Card (PRC).

Remember to visit **www.innatechiro.com** to download and print your own copy of the PRC.

I have been using the Personal Report Card (PRC) in my office since 2012. I have found it to be a great tool to assess a patient's habits and see how they progress over time. The eleven categories I choose to grade are the best habits or attributes that the healthiest and happiest people most commonly have As in.

How to Give Yourself a Grade

We all remember getting grades in school, and my report card is not much different than that. However, the emphasis is on improving your health, not passing English. With this tool, your health is like your GPA—except, in this case, it's your *Health Point Average* (HPA). There is actually a simple HPA tool on my website. When you are done filling out your report card, check it out and get your overall HPA at **www.innatechiro.com**. You'll also find a blank report card that you can print out so you can fill out a new one whenever you want.

PERSONAL REPORT CARD

Name: _____   Date: _____

HEALTH MARKERS	GRADE			ACTION STEPS
	Current	Goal	Goal Date	
Diet				
Supplementation				
Exercise				
Body Composition				
Sleep				
Hydration				
Alignment/Posture				
Stress Management				
Connectedness				
Health Awareness				
Elimination				

Notes:

Here are the primary topic areas I grade patients on:

1. *Diet*
2. *Supplementation*
3. *Exercise*
4. *Body Composition:* your percentage of muscle compared to fat
5. *Sleep:* quantity and quality
6. *Hydration:* Are you getting enough water?
7. *Alignment and Posture:* How do you carry yourself?
8. *Stress Management:* How well do you handle stress?
9. *Connectedness:* spending time connecting to self and/or a higher power
10. *Health Awareness:* How much time do you spend learning about heath?
11. *Elimination:* bowel movements

Here's how to fill out your first report card:

Picture yourself as the head teacher for a student. The student, of course, is you. Let's start with the first category, *Diet.* What grade would you give yourself if someone asked you how great your overall diet was? Would you give yourself an A? Are you more like a C+? The grade you give yourself is very subjective. What that means is that it's based upon opinion. *Your* opinion of the quality of your overall diet. Not sure what grade to give yourself? You can use the guidelines listed in the upcoming pages for some reference points for grades, but you don't *really* need them. Just picture what your idea of the greatest diet on the planet would be and make that an A. How does the way you eat right now measure up to it?

Do the same thing for the other subjects. Let's use exercise. Can you picture how often, how intense, and what type of exercise regimen would get you an A? Are you already there? Remember, this is simply your opinion. If you believe that walking twenty to thirty minutes a day is an A and that's what you do, then give yourself an A. If you believe that you don't have an A unless you can complete an Ironman Triathlon in under fourteen hours, then grade yourself on that scale. I'm simply asking you to take a few minutes and measure where *you* think *you* are when it comes to the most important healthy habits and attributes.

Go ahead and fill out your report card! Do it in pencil for now, and as you keep reading, if you feel that you want to change your grade, go ahead. I review report cards with my patients once to twice a year depending on how often I see them and what they're working on.

Below are some guidelines on how to grade yourself in each of the areas. You can base your grading system on these guidelines, alter them to be at a "competitive athlete" level, or alter them to be just slightly better than where you are right now. I'll go into detail about each of the areas throughout the remainder of the book. Keep reading to get the most out of your PRC!

Dr. Piken's Grading System Guidelines

Diet

This is the most challenging area to give guidelines for because there are so many different diets that work for different people. Here are some general guidelines to receive an A grade. Make sure to consult the help of a nutritionist to find out your personal optimal diet and create your own grade guidelines for A through D!

A

I eat four to six small meals a day.

I eat seven to nine servings of fruits and veggies (mostly vegetables).

One-third of the food I eat is raw food, or I eat at least one salad a day.

I avoid all foods that make me bloat or cause digestive upset.

I eat mostly organic foods.

I eat no more than I need to maintain my muscle percentage goals.

B

I eat three to four times a day.

I eat great during the week but "eat whatever I want on the weekends."

I read labels on the foods I buy, and I try to make better choices.

In general, my weight doesn't fluctuate much because my diet is consistent.

C

My choices match those of a B, but I overeat and see my weight creeping up slowly but surely.

D

I often eat fast food.

I often feel bloated from food.

I'm not getting closer to my muscle percentage goals.

I eat a lot of processed/convenience foods.

Supplementation

A

I have a doctor/nutritionist who has recommended a program for me.

I'm diligent about taking recommended supplements daily.

B

I have figured out what I need from articles online, and I take my supplements most days.

C

I have a great multivitamin and a fish oil supplement, and I take them one to three times a week.

D

I have an inexpensive multivitamin I got at the supermarket, and I take it "when I remember."

Exercise

Again, an A here will be different for a competitive athlete compared to someone just starting to work out. The suggestions below are flexible. What I like to do with patients when working on their report card is to ask them what they think optimal exercise means to them, then base the grades on where they currently are. Here are some suggestions.

A

I'm physically active six times a week with a mix of strength, flexibility, and aerobic training. I'm physically active at least three times a week with moderate to intense exercise.

B

I'm physically active three times a week. I only do one type of exercise with the same routine each time.

C

I'm physically active one to two times a week.

I walk to the office and back home, fifteen to twenty minutes each way.

Body Composition

For a body composition grade, you first need to find a good way to get an accurate measurement of your body fat/muscle percentage. The industry standard is a dual-energy X-ray absorptiometry (DEXA) study or water immersion study, but you can get a fairly accurate reading from different types of bioelectrical impedance analysis machines, which you can find at many health-focused doctors' offices. In my office, we use a unit that measures you electronically by sending a microcurrent from your hand to your foot. It is much more accurate than hand-to-hand only devices or the devices that you stand on that measure foot to foot.

Below is a chart of optimal percentages of muscle depending on your age range. Simply subtract the number below from one hundred to figure out what your optimal body fat percentage should be.

Muscle Percentage[1]

AGE

MALES		15-24	25-34	35-44	45-54	55-64	65-74	75-84	>85
	A	88.4%	84.8%	82.4%	80.3%	77.8%	75.4%	73.7%	68.6%
	B	86.4%	82.8%	80.4%	78.3%	75.8%	73.4%	71.7%	66.6%
	C	83.4%	79.8%	77.4%	75.3%	72.8%	70.4%	68.7%	63.6%
	D	80.4%	76.8%	74.4%	72.3%	69.8%	67.4%	65.7%	60.6%

AGE

FEMALES		15-24	25-34	35-44	45-54	55-64	65-74	75-84	>85
	A	78.4%	77.5%	76.1%	74.2%	70.9%	65.7%	64.2%	62.4%
	B	76.4%	75.5%	74.1%	72.2%	68.9%	63.7%	62.2%	60.4%
	C	73.4%	72.5%	71.1%	69.2%	65.9%	60.7%	59.2%	57.4%
	D	70.4%	69.5%	68.1%	66.2%	62.9%	57.7%	56.2%	54.4%

[1] A Values taken from: Kyle UG, et al. "Fat-Free and Fat Mass Percentiles in 5225 Healthy Subjects Aged 15 to 98 Years." Nutrition, 17:534–541, 2001.

ALTERNATIVE BODY COMPOSITION GRADING GUIDELINES

Simply go with how you look and feel. A great place to start is your belly.

A++

Eight-pack

A+

Six-pack

A

Flat belly (naturally ... not sucked in)

B

Belly sticks out a bit

C

Overweight

D

Obese

F

Morbidly obese (lack of muscle impacting daily life and health)

You can also use your body mass index (BMI). It's a simple tool that gives you a number grade based on your height and weight. I don't love it because it has flaws, but if you need some type of reference to start with, it is accurate often. The biggest flaws come from people that have atypical height-to-weight ratios like bodybuilders or some very petite-framed people.

A

BMI between 18–22

B

BMI between 23–26

C

BMI between 27–30

D

BMI between 31–34

F

BMI above 34

Please refer to the BMI chart in the Appendix to calculate your BMI.

Sleep

A

I get seven and a half to eight and a half hours of restful sleep per night on average.

B

I get six to seven hours of restful sleep per night on average.

C

I get six hours of restful sleep per night on average, but I have trouble falling asleep and/or staying asleep.

D

I get under six hours of restful sleep per night on average.

Hydration

A

I'm not often very thirsty.
I tend to drink about half my weight in fluid ounces of water daily (see Chapter 13).

B

I drink water often, yet I also feel thirsty often. (Hint... . Think about evaluating your blood sugar and/or electrolyte consumption and digestion—see the chapter on hydration for more on this.)

C

I only drink water when I'm really thirsty.
I drink colas or fruit drinks often.

D

Um, does beer count towards hydration?

Alignment and Posture

A

I carry myself in a way that is proud, tall, energetic, and symmetrical!

B

All of the above applies to me, but one shoulder is higher than the other, my head sticks out too far forward, or I slouch at work.

C

I am a frequent sloucher with lots of asymmetry due to many years of slouching.

D

I am someone who passes a chiropractor at a health fair and cringes because I know my posture is horrible.

Stress Management

A

Even when life is stressful, I handle it with ease.

B

I worry or get depressed from time to time.

C

I am frequently worried, anxious, or stressed out.

D

I need medication and/or therapy to be able to cope with the stresses of life.

F

You can find me curled up in a ball under the covers.

Connectedness

Are you doing something every day to disconnect from the electronic world and connect with yourself and the people around you? Here are the guidelines I use to keep myself connected.

A

I practice meditation for twenty minutes twice a day
I practice journaling each night.
I follow all the B-grade guidelines as well.

B

I practice daily prayer and create a gratitude list.
I practice meditation for ten to fifteen minutes most days.
I read positive books.
I follow all the C-grade guidelines as well.

C

I take long walks with my dog or I just walk and think two to three times a week.
I practice daily breathing exercises for five minutes a day.

D

I use meditation or an alternative stress management method in an effort to "get connected" when stressed, but it is a reactive effort as opposed to a proactive daily practice.

F

I escape frequently with TV, alcohol, or video games (it's fine to "escape" sometimes, as long as you can fit in your escape *after* you've established and completed your connection time).

Health Awareness

How knowledgeable are you on the topic of health? If you don't know how to care for yourself, then you'll simply keep doing what you've always done. Or maybe you jump from one health tip to the other. We all need to have at least a basic understanding of how the human body works and how to care for it. An important part of improving your health and quality of life is improving your mindset and level of health awareness. The following are the guidelines I use.

A

I read articles/blogs/books or listen to podcasts about health and life improvement every day.

B

I read articles/blogs/books or listen to podcasts about health and life improvement once or twice a week

C

I try to learn something at doctor visits.

D

I get health info from friends, celebrity magazines, or from the thirty-second clip at the end of the news.

F

I'm very passive; I expect the doctors to take care of things.

Elimination

A simple way to evaluate elimination is by studying your poop. Yes, this is very crude, but it does give you some insight into how your body deals with eliminating toxins.

A

I poop one to three times a day.
All my bowel movements look like well-formed logs, and there is no strain.

B

I poop daily, but the consistency of the movement changes based on what I eat.
I notice undigested food occasionally.

The consistency can be a little soft, or the log can consist of many little balls.

C–D

I poop infrequently or too frequently.
The consistency is poor.
A grade of C or D can also include:

- Constipation: I have bowel movements one to five times a week, and I feel like I still need to evacuate more after a movement. The poop is dry and/or has the consistency of little balls.
- Loose Stool: I have bowel movements two to five times a day that are not well-formed. They can range from a toothpaste-like consistency to watery.

D–F

IBS pattern (irritable bowel syndrome)
There is no rhyme or reason to my poop schedule or consistency.

For the most part in these guidelines, I've just given you what A, B, C, and D grades look like. At times, I've added a description for an F. When creating your grading guidelines, you can add in what a (+) and (–) would look like, too. For example, what would a B+ look like as opposed to a B? What would an A+ look like in each area? Don't be afraid to be as specific as possible. The more specific you are, the more precise you can be with your self-assessments while you're grading yourself. It will also be easier to see and track your progress. You'll be able to celebrate more increments of progress along the way as you improve each of these areas.

Okay. Now is the time to go create your grading guidelines for yourself. Get something down for each section—you can evolve your guidelines as you read through this book and get inspired. The important thing is to get something down now for each area. You can create your PRC however you want. You can write out your guidelines at the beginning of a notebook and simply write out each area and the grade you're giving yourself each time you do a report. Or you could create your PRC on the computer so you can print out several copies and easily fill in the grades each time you reassess yourself. Head over to my website www.innatechiro.com to print out more report cards for yourself and you can also enter your grades into the Health Point Average Calculator. You could make a colorful visual display on paperboard with inspiring pictures and quotes. Use whatever format you prefer. The most important part is that you create it!

Next, give yourself your first grades for each of the areas. Congratulations! Now you have your starting point.

Chapter 4

Setting
Your Goals

Now that you've created your PRC and have filled in your current grades, let's focus on where you want to go! Let's say you have a C+ diet—do you really want to be an A+? Would a B+ be great? Maybe simply moving to a B is a great goal until your next report card. No matter what your goal is—no matter how small or how big—please make sure it's *really what you want*!

Think of it this way: I would really love eight-pack abs, compete on *American Ninja Warrior* and climb the big warped wall and hit the buzzer, and I would really love to complete an Ironman Triathlon ... but I *don't* want to invest the time it would take to actually accomplish these goals. If I put them on my list of goals but feel bad about spending time away from my family, my professional practice, my time learning more about health, and my time walking my dogs—and if I'm unhappy because I have to watch every bite of food I eat—then I will be conflicted and therefore not really focused on what I want. In other words, I may want to reach these goals, but I am distracted by other things that I also want. It's important to me to have amazing relationships with my wife and kids and to spend a few hours a week learning. I could have all of these things if I planned out every second of my day as such, but I would have to be losing sleep, and proper sleep is also important to me. I love to get seven to eight hours of sleep every day.

My report card goals take into account *all* aspects of my life. If I really want to improve my HPA but believe I can *only* get an A in *Exercise* if I'm cycling twenty miles a day and swimming a mile a day, then I'm probably going to have to alter my definition of what an A is for me. For me personally, right now, an A is moderate to intense exercise at least three times a week and being physically active in some way (yoga, hiking, golf, or a light jog) on the other days. I want to challenge my body a little bit every day. That's my A. What's yours? Make sure your As in each area fit your goals in all aspects of your life, meaning you don't have to make big sacrifices in one important area of your life to score achievements in another.

What if you think you have straight As? If you have straight As, then great! You've already achieved optimum growth—but take a look to see if you actually want to knock your As down to Bs or B pluses to give yourself room to reach an even better grade.

If you really feel like you are getting straight As, or even As, then I would say it's time for you to share this by teaching. Once you have achieved your own personal optimum growth, there is nothing that will make you feel better than sharing your techniques of how you did it and helping others grow, just as you did. But why not still also give yourself some room to grow? Growing is one of the most fulfilling things we can do as human beings. It feels great to see ourselves become better than we were before. So even if you've reached your optimum level in some areas, push yourself to grow in others. Challenge yourself to keep getting better and better. Growth makes for a healthy, happy life.

Chapter 5

Redefining Your Rules

What good is health if you're miserable following all of the rules? It depends on your goals and who you ask. Did John Belushi, Chris Farley, Jimi Hendrix, Marilyn Monroe, and Amy Winehouse live the right way? These are all examples of people who lived fast, hard lives filled with excess. I bet if you asked their family and close friends, they would say they messed it all up. Some fans may say they lived life fast and hard and went out playing their own game and following their own rules. You might say that underlying depression or immaturity played a part in their tragic, early deaths. You might also say that none of us would have ever heard of any of them if they hadn't lived the way they had.

My first associate, Dr. Andreas Clironomos, once shared a thought with me that has stuck with me ever since. When I hired him, I was definitely *not* ready for an associate. I wasn't prepared to take on the task of basically running an apprenticeship in my office when I really had not even scratched the surface of what it takes to grow into the leader a team. I was unorganized, and my practice wasn't set up for anyone but myself. I only knew how to attract the Dr. Piken patients, and I had absolutely no idea how to attract the Dr. Clironomos patients. Luckily, I had hired someone who realized this, and after three weeks, we had a talk that led to him finding a job at another office a few blocks away that was a better place for him to grow. He had a great heart, and I was happy for him.

During our first sit-down, he said something very simple yet very enlightening. This twenty-something philosopher said, "Jason, life is just like a game, and we all choose to play it differently. Some of us will cheat, some will be fair, some will make few alliances, some will ask for help, and some will be leaders. However, *you* choose to play this game—and it's all just a game—it's the game of life." I did paraphrase and maybe add a bit in there, but this thought has stuck with me ever since.

I can't say that I didn't already know this deep down inside, but up until that point, I had never heard it worded in that particular way. Nobody is playing the game wrong. We all think that our version of the game is right. That's what's so fascinating about humans, groups, families, clubs, religions, etc.—everyone thinks they're right. In my opinion, as long as you don't try to force *your* views of this game onto *other* people, then you're okay. I may not agree with your philosophy. I may think that your version of the game is downright ridiculous. But as long as your game doesn't interfere with mine, then it works for me.

This tenet should be understood by all. It would solve most of the world's biggest problems if we all followed it. Life is a game, and we all play it differently. Let everyone else play their own game of life, unless their game harms others. That's a universal rule—to live and let live: Play the game however you like, but as soon as your game starts to interfere with someone else's, leave them alone and let them play the way they want to play. This applies regardless of how strongly you believe everyone else should be playing the game *your* way, your group's way, or your religion's way.

If you educate a person who isn't playing the game "correctly" and they choose to play the game their way, I believe it's best to just let them be. You may attempt to try "saving" them through teaching peacefully, but as soon as they make it clear that they do *not* want to play the game the same way you do, let them be. It's unlikely that their decision will harm you or anyone else. They may be trampling on your beliefs and what you know to be true, but unless there is real evidence that their game is harming you and your life, then simply *let it be!*

Think of all the religious squabbles that could be resolved if we all just chose to play our own games like this. Think of the level of understanding we could all have—and the ability to move on—if we just accepted each other's choices and continued focusing on our own games of life.

The beautiful thing is that we can always change the way we play *our* games. If you learn something or are enlightened by the way someone else is living, you can adjust how you live. Join their team or copy the way they play. It's still a *game*, and the greatest part of this game is that *you make your own rules.* You could choose to play like John Belushi, or you could choose to play like Gandhi. You could choose to play like Reverend Jerry Falwell, like Tony Robbins, or like your buddy Gregg down the block.

If you see someone who you don't think is playing the game in the best way, stop and educate them. Try to teach them and pour your heart into it, but accept it if they still choose to play the game their own way in the end.

There are also rules for the society you live in. For example, if you're playing your game and you notice someone is lying, cheating, stealing, or harming others in some way, then as a member of the same society, you can call them out. I believe that's another universal rule: *the Golden Rule*—treat others as you wish to be treated. As long as you inform the authorities at hand when you notice someone is breaking

DR. JASON PIKEN • BETTER!

this rule, we can all keep playing our moral version of the game in our own ways.

Think about the game of life that *you* want to play. What are some of your rules? What rules would enable you to reach the point you want in your life in terms of health and happiness? In this book, I present you with my rules for living a healthy, happy life. In the next section, we'll talk about how to turn some of those rules into habits, so you can start benefiting from them!

> **RULE:**
>
> Make your own rules that work for *you*.

REPORT CARD REFECTION TIME:

After reading a bit more, how do you feel about your initial grades on your report card? I recommended that you fill it out for the first time in pencil so you can change your grades if you want. Sit back with your report card for a few minutes and evaluate the grades you really want to give yourself now. Don't worry about getting it wrong. There is no right or wrong. This is your personal opinion of how you're doing. As you keep learning more, your opinion will change. In the next sections, you'll learn how to improve your grades in all of the categories!

PART III

Setting Yourself
Up for Success

Chapter 6

Establishing Rituals and Healthy Habits

Now that we've talked about rules—and how *your rules* are based on the game of life that *you* want to play— let's talk about *rituals* and *habits*.

When you know what kind of life you want to live, you can make sure that you're able to live that life by establishing habits that are consistent with it. Your report card will let you know how you're doing and whether or not you're getting closer to the life you want. For example, let's say you gave yourself a C grade in *Exercise*, and you want to get to a B+ by your next report card. Maybe you gave yourself a C because you have a gym membership but you only go to the gym in spurts. Over the course of a month, you get there five to eight times—sometimes two to three times a week and other weeks, not at all.

The first thing you have to imagine is exactly what a B+ looks like as far as your lifestyle goes. Let's say that in order to get to a B+, you decide that getting to the gym three times every week is a must. Next, you determine a minimum length of time you would need to spend at the gym on each visit—let's say it's twenty-five minutes. So now you understand that someone who is a B+ in *Exercise*, in your mind, is someone who goes to the gym three times each week for a minimum of twenty-five minutes each time. Great! Now you have your goal. These then become the habits that you need to develop in order to bring up your mark. Start tracking right away. A week, to me, begins on Monday and ends on Sunday, so if Friday comes around and you haven't made it to the gym yet, then you're going Friday, Saturday, and Sunday so you don't blow your grade!

I wish I had a magic formula for setting grades and goals for you, but it's simply impossible. We're all different people with different situations and ways of viewing the world. The point of coming up with your own grades, your own goals, and the habits and rituals that will get you there is to sit down and work it all out for yourself. It's the only way to do it. We tend to learn best from our own experiences and, often, our own mistakes. If we're simply told what to do, we may follow directions for a short period of time, but when we create our *own* rules and habits based on our own personal desires and goals, I believe that they're much more powerful. It's like that proverb by Lao Tzu: *Give a man a fish and you feed him for a day. Teach a man to fish and you feed him for a lifetime.*

The key to improving your scores on your PRC is creating healthy habits that enable you to improve each area, bit by bit. Improvements don't just happen by doing something once. Improvement in any area of your life follows after doing something over and over until it becomes a habit.

If you're really passionate about your new habits, then you can even take them to the next level: *rituals.* Let me give you an example. Brushing my teeth daily is a habit that will never be a ritual. I do it because I *have* to—not because I thoroughly enjoy it. Sure, it feels good to get that taste out of your mouth in the morning or after some meals, but I just don't get great joy out of this two-minute habit. Now, on the other hand, let's talk about my *Grateful* list! Each morning, I write down three to seven things that I'm grateful for in a journal that I keep. This has become a ritual for me…. Let me describe it!

At first, the task of doing this was assigned to me by my coach—notice the words used there: *task* and *assigned*. At the time, I felt that I already had enough things to get done in the morning, so I didn't want to add anything else in. However, I had been paying a coach a nice amount of money to push me in the right direction to help me get where I wanted to be, so I implemented this task as told. Each day I would think about three to seven things that I was grateful for while lying in bed each morning, and then I would get out of bed and start my day. I didn't get that much out of it, but it was a nice exercise that became a habit.

I had been doing this for a few months before my coach realized that I wasn't following the rules. You see, he had told me to *write down* three to seven things I was grateful for each day. When I learned that what I was doing wasn't "good enough," I was, of course, annoyed at first because now I had to suffer through the *tremendous ordeal* of getting out of bed and having a pen and paper ready to write my grateful list each morning. But I was a diligent student, and I had the motivation to make my life better, so I listened.

That was when the habit changed for me. There's something magical about writing things down. We're losing the experience in the modern age because we're typing everything on keyboards, but there really is something nice about pen on paper—you get to see your thoughts materialize into words on paper. That's when my daily habit developed into a *ritual*. I enjoy seeing the words. Words like:

I am grateful for the hugs my daughters gave me when I came home from work last night.

I am grateful that my wife cares for her body and looks really good because of it.

I am grateful that I had time to walk my dogs yesterday.

I am grateful that my office team was inspired to do better after our weekly training yesterday.

I am grateful for hot water on a cold day.

This is the reason it became a ritual. A ritual is more than a habit that you perform each day. It becomes a ritual when it has a deep meaning or makes you feel especially good every time you do it. For some, it's the ritual of prayer. For others, it's exercise.

I got a similar feeling while I was typing the words for this book, but I'll tell you, not as much as pen to paper. Maybe it's a generational thing—you may get the same feeling by typing—but I will challenge you to try writing a grateful list on paper first. For me, it became a *ritual* rather than a chore or simply a habit because after doing it, I feel better—and after doing it now for many years, I *look forward to it*.

The PRC is a tool to help you take an honest look at your habits and see which ones you need to upgrade or change. Take a look at the PRC grades you just gave yourself. Can you already see areas where you need to create new habits? Can you envision any of these turning into rituals?

The Four-Month Rule

Let's talk a little more about *creating* habits. How do you create a new habit? First, you have to look ahead and plan out four months in front of you. Set yourself up to be able to implement your new habit for four months. If you can't keep up a change for at least four months, you haven't made a change at all! Implementing something new for any less amount of time than that is just a temporary phase.

Let's take the process I outlined a few paragraphs ago, for example. Let's say your goal is to work out three times a week for twenty-five minutes a day, minimum. The first thing you have to do is make it through four months, or else you really haven't created enough momentum to keep you going. The hardest part of implementing any new habit is the first three weeks. If you can make it through the first three weeks without any excuses, then the fourth week will be a little easier, the fifth week even easier, and so on.

Throughout the four months, you're still going to have little struggles, but challenge yourself to keep up that habit of exercising three times a week, even if it's merely fifteen minutes one day, thirty minutes the next, and sixty-five minutes the next—it's still twenty-five minutes a day on average. And, the most important thing is that you show up three times a week. If you can keep it up for four months, you create so much momentum that it would become hard to break the habit. It's becomes harder to stop than to keep going! Remember—three times a week for four months. *No excuses*!

Think about what your life was like four months ago. It doesn't seem like that long ago, right? Now imagine if you had been doing something to achieve your goals on a regular basis for the last four months. Would you miss the time you spent on your phone crushing candy or your time on Facebook and Instagram? Wouldn't it be nice to look back four months and reflect on the time and effort you invested in being proud of yourself and have a feeling of accomplishment? Just start *now* and make yourself better!

Make something better! In time, the *real* goal is to get this habit to last the rest of your life because it's a healthy habit that you'd never want to give up. Start with something now!

QUICK TIP: Stick It on Your Mirror!

Do you have a bathroom mirror? I bet you do! I hope you do! If there's one thing you want to change right now and you want it to last the next

four months—and then forever—write it down on a Post-It note or grab a nice piece of paper and write down exactly what you're going to do for the next four months. You look at that mirror at least a couple of times a day, so it will be a constant reminder. Don't simply ignore it, though… . You have to read it every time you see it. No matter how sick of it you get, just keep reading the statement to yourself; out loud would be even better!

Earlier, I mentioned that guy Gregg down the block. Here's what his note stated. He taped it to his bathroom mirror!

> I will exercise for at least twenty minutes a day and at least three times a week I will do this without fail at least until October 22.

👍 QUICK TIP: Anchoring Habits

I have a great tip for developing new habits: Anchor them to habits you already practice. For example, brushing your teeth. Most of us brush our teeth at least once per day, hopefully twice and maybe even three times. This is already an anchored habit—something we do every single day of our lives without fail. If we want to remember to introduce another habit, anchor it to one that's already solid … like brushing your teeth. It doesn't necessarily have to be anchored to brushing your teeth—if you have another solid habit that you do every single day, anchor it to that—I just use brushing your teeth as an example. We usually have routines before going to bed as well, so these routines are good ones to attach new habits to as well, if brushing your teeth isn't a regular practice before bed.

As soon as you finish brushing your teeth (or whatever habit you're going to use as the anchor), start your new habit! You don't have to do the new habit immediately, but brushing your teeth should be a *trigger* for thinking about exactly when you will complete your new habit that day. Let me give you the example of a patient of mine. Let's call her Robin.

Robin just could not remember to take her supplements that she was supposed to be taking. She took them sometimes, *when she remembered*. Robin was supposed to take her supplements twice per day at breakfast and lunch, but she told me she was too busy and distracted. Here's what I had her do. First, I reminded her of her *whys*: She was achy and stiff in the morning getting out of bed, she felt she didn't handle stress well, and she frequently caught colds in the winter. I asked Robin where she ate breakfast. She ate breakfast at a small table in her kitchen. I asked her where she ate lunch. During the week, it was at her desk at work. I then asked her where she kept her supplements. In a cabinet in her kitchen, she replied. Can you picture how she could remember to take her supplements better? Can you picture her anchors? I simply had Robin keep her morning supplements in the center of the little breakfast table and her afternoon supplements on her desk at work. Sure, she complained that the supplements would annoy her, being out in the open like that. They didn't look nice. I simply told her to deal with it for four months until she was used to taking her supplements along with breakfast and lunch.

Guess what? Robin has fewer colds, handles stress better, and is less achy in the morning. She kept her supplements out in the open because she didn't mind the tradeoff. Robin realized it was better to alter her habits and feel better than to stick with an old set of rules (supplements belong on the shelf in a cabinet) that kept her from changing.

Lunch is a great anchor point—whenever you think of having lunch, anchor your new habit then, whether that's taking supplements, doing a midday meditation, exercising, or doing some reading. See how easy it is to anchor your new habits to other habits you already have?

Let's say one of your goals is to get rid of sore gums and frequent cavities, and your health professional has recommended a few supplements you should take daily to improve your diet. While you're brushing your teeth, read your goal sheet to remind yourself why you should take your supplements, and think about the delicious vegetables you're going to put in your salad at lunch. You can use the trigger of brushing your teeth to prompt you to plan how to fulfill your other habits as well. By planning exactly how you're going to accomplish your daily health habits, you are much more likely to do them. You simply have to prioritize the habits you want to accomplish. It's worth also noting here that ultimately, the things that we make our highest priority are the new habits we are successful at implementing.

What are some daily tasks that you can anchor onto? If it's not brushing your teeth, is there something better? Take a minute to think about it and write a note right here on the side of the book! To be successful in implementing new habits, anchor them to simple, everyday tasks. When you do this, you'll be surprised at how easy it is to keep them up!

> **RULE:**
>
> Anchor your rules to daily tasks so you remember to do them!

Increase the Good! (Don't Just Decrease the Bad)

This should be a motto for how you are going to change your life for the better. Many people find it really difficult to accomplish the following:

- Lose weight
- Give up coffee
- Give up chocolate
- Stop eating fast food
- Limit TV to one hour a day
- Stop eating starchy, sweet foods

One of the ways I motivate people to make changes is to get them add more goodness into their lives. If you keep adding good into your life, there automatically won't be as much room for the bad. When it comes to keeping up new habits, people have much higher success rates by adding in more good stuff than focusing on doing less of the bad.

Reducing negative habits is restrictive and involves immense willpower. It can be done, but it's based on how much discipline you have with yourself—there's lots of room to slip. Thinking about taking things away often doesn't feel good. On the other hand, adding in more good things allows you to reach for what you want. You're focused on where you're going. It's way more fun, and it feels good. And you're keeping a promise to yourself at the same time.

Here are some examples of how to increase more good:

- Eat two medium-sized carrots every day before you leave the house

  Benefits: Increases fiber intake, increases nutrient intake, fills you with real food instead of crap, and helps you avoid skipping a meal with a simple daily activity

- Wake up twenty minutes earlier

  Benefits: Enables more time to meditate/exercise, eliminates rushing around and getting stressed before work

- Eat a salad every day for lunch

  Benefits: Prevents you from falling for foods that you crave due to stress, increases veggie consumption, increases raw food intake, increases fiber, contains fewer calories than the lunch you're eating now

- Have vegetables with pasta, not pasta with vegetables

- It's a play on words, but it does make a difference—if you're not ready to give up your pasta, then make sure you eat a giant amount of vegetables *with* your pasta. Most restaurants portion vegetables as a side dish. The ratio of vegetables to pasta in my meals at home is three to one, vegetables to pasta—not the other way around.

  Benefits: Too many to list here!

- Exercise—add in even just ten minutes a day

- Meditate—add in just ten minutes a day

- Journal—again, add in just ten minutes a day

If you just add these last three rules into your life, then you have just added half an hour of additional quality, positive things to your life. This is time you would have most likely spent doing something unhealthy, and now you've replaced it with greatness!

If you keep working on making positive changes to your life by putting in more good foods and making more time in your day for positive habits, then you can't help but displace the unhealthy habits because you'll no longer have time for them.

> **RULE:**
>
> Add one new good food or positive habit into your life every few weeks until your grade is better.

Stop It!

While the key is to focus on adding more good, not taking out the bad, sometimes there are things that you simply need to *stop doing*. For example, eating starchy foods, gossiping, eating late at night, and eating foods that bloat you. As such, I had to add a small section here about how to stop doing things that are no longer serving you. But it's the shortest chapter in the book!

I simply must recommend that you do an Internet search for: "Stop It! / Bob Newhart." It's a hilarious skit that explains, with great eloquence, what we need to do anytime we want to make a change in our lives. Do it now! Put down the book for six to seven minutes, get on your phone or computer, and watch one of the best skits out there on changing habits!

> **RULE:**
>
> Stop. Take out things that are not serving you anymore.

Do Not Try to Do Anything; Decide to Do Something!

When you're faced with the choice of acting out a healthy habit or an unhealthy habit, make the decision to go with the healthy habit and cut off all other options. Once you've made a decision to do something, you are so much more at ease with it than if you *try* to do something; for example, "I'm going to *try* to avoid desert," or "I'm going to *try* to go to the gym this week." As soon as you put the word *try* in the sentence, you've already given yourself an out! As you're reading, you may be realizing there are many habits in your life you want to change. You may not be able to do everything right now. Start by determining the *most important* change you need to make in your life (the one that will impact your report card the most) and *decide* that you are going to do it!

Make promises to yourself! I don't make promises to myself very often. The reason for this is that once I decide to do something and make a promise to myself, *I follow through and do it*. Sometimes that scares me, so I won't make a promise to myself that I'm scared of following through with or one that concerns me. Once the promise is made, I don't go back on it.

Here's a great example: I decided to live gluten-free to see how I felt. What is gluten? Gluten is a protein found in wheat, rye, and barley products that can cause inflammation if your body is sensitive or allergic to it (more on food sensitivities at the Special Circumstances section). I've learned so much about how gluten can ruin some people's lives. Lab testing in New York is not always conclusive, however, especially if you only have a sensitivity rather than a full-blown allergy, so if you suspect that gluten is causing issues in your body, it's best to avoid eating it altogether for at least three months to see how it affects you. I decided to go gluten free at a seminar after hearing, once again, that I needed to try it. I knew it was an all-or-nothing proposition. Living gluten-free is not a simple thing to do. There's wheat everywhere! No more pizza or pasta or fried calamari. But I was ready! From that day on, I was gluten free.

At the time, I knew I needed ninety days to get a good evaluation, so I committed to ninety days. Here's a great tip: When making a decision that will change your habits, give yourself a *definitive time frame* in which you will make the change without any excuses. I began this ninety-day period of eating gluten free a couple weeks before Thanksgiving, which usually would mean that it wasn't a "good time" to do it. But when is it really a good time to make a habit change? The answer is, *whenever you're ready*. I was gluten-free through Thanksgiving, my daughter's birthday, Chanukah, Christmas, an all-inclusive vacation to St. Thomas (where I had to choose from whatever they had), New Year's Eve, and a Super Bowl party. These major events during those ninety days could have easily represented "not a good time," but I was *ready*! And, it was *easy*!

It was easy because I made a decision, and a decision to me means I've cut off all other options. I decided that, to me, eating gluten was the equivalent of eating cockroaches. Sure, I was tempted by the things I had been eating freely just a few days or weeks before. Sure, it would have been even easier if I had noticed an immediate difference and felt any better, but I didn't notice a single change in my life as a result of cutting out gluten. However, I stuck to it anyway because I had made one of those promises to *myself*. I noticed no change after reintroducing gluten back into my life. I did love that gigantic bowl of pasta and fresh-baked bakery bread from the Bronx, though. I still don't consider the experiment a waste, however, because I learned something. I learned that I can keep a promise to myself. It always feels great when you set a goal to do something and you actually follow through with it.

By the way, now, after running the diagnostic genetic tests for celiac disease on myself, I have again begun living gluten free. Celiac disease is a genetic allergy or intolerance to gluten. A positive genetic test doesn't necessarily mean that you will become symptomatic. In any case, I find that I eat much better when I have certain limiting rules, so I am heeding my genetic warning signal. I'm hoping that it will make me feel better in some way, but this time I'm giving myself a year, not ninety days ... and *yes*, it's easy this time but only because, again, I made a decision—there's no other option in my mind!

> **RULE:**
>
> Don't *try* anything. If you want something to change, make a *decision* to change it *now*! Set a time limit for how long you will carry out the change. Don't make any promises to yourself that you can't keep!

Chapter 7

Creating a Great Morning Routine

Get an Early Start to the Day

How you set up your day is key in making sure you set yourself up for success. Without a great morning routine, it will be tough to implement any changes that will improve the areas of your report card. Every day you live starts with your morning. So we're going to establish some rules about yours.

For the vast majority of my life, prior to about age twenty-nine, I was *not* a morning person. There are pictures in my high school yearbook of me sleeping on a desk in the middle of class. I was actually a great student, but I just could not stay awake most of the day. In college, I tried my hardest to avoid classes that began before noon, and this usually worked. I even took a few night classes with the Adult Ed department so I wouldn't have to wake up early or have to try to pay attention before noon.

My wife turned me into a morning person, and I am incredibly glad she did. One of my rules now is to wake up and start the day early—as the saying goes, "Early to bed and early to rise... ." This might not work if you're a bartender, a waiter in the catering business, or a musician, of course. There are many exceptions, but for the most part, we are a nation of daytime work and activity. If you're in this category, then wake up earlier. You will get so many more things accomplished. You'll also have better quality sleep because our circadian rhythms—our bodies' internal time clocks—naturally want us to wake up early and go to bed early.

I'll never forget my turnaround day. I can still remember the emotions and a lot of the activities of that day because it had such a major impact on how I organize my life today. My wife was always a morning person. During our first few years as a couple, I remember her being up for hours on a Saturday—running errands, going for walks, shopping, and eating breakfast—then coming home to her husband who was still in bed at noon, sleeping like a log. It must have been frustrating. She comes from a family of early-risers. For years, her dad used to wake up at 4:30 a.m. to work out with his trainer before starting his day. One day, my wife asked me to try it her way. She proposed that the following Saturday, we would wake up at a reasonable hour—at 8 a.m.—and start our day. I was up for it—at least for just one day.

I still remember her standing over me in bed that Saturday morning. I must have pulled the covers over my head to just get a few extra minutes of sleep, hoping that she'd forget about the whole thing. But she didn't forget. I didn't fight much because a promise is a promise, so we got up, and I showered and got dressed. We walked up the block and had breakfast at *Tal Bagels, the best bagel place in NYC*— a place that, nowadays, make me really miss gluten. We took a ride down to Soho, shopped, and walked around, enjoying a beautiful summer day in the city. She wanted to shop a bit more and I went along with her, even though I hate shopping for more than ten minutes per store. This was her day, so I did it, and I actually ended up getting a few things I needed.

We got back to the apartment and I plopped onto the couch to pass out for a bit, exhausted. Suddenly, I sat up, startled. "*Oh no...* . I'm wiping out, and we have to go to dinner with friends tonight... . How will I make it?"

I quickly asked Stacey what time it was, and she told me that it was 2 p.m.

Only 2 p.m.! This meant I still had six hours before I needed to get ready for dinner. I had had the equivalent of a full day, which had been fun and also productive, and I could nap for two to three hours, wake up, go to the gym, and still have enough time to relax before dinner. I was *sold*! This was so much better than the Saturday before had been, as well as most of my Saturdays, which typically consisted of sleeping for ten hours until 1 p.m., getting up, and feeling really lazy. After that, most of the day would consist of lying around in bed, watching TV, ordering food to be delivered so I didn't have to leave my bed, and procrastinating until reaching a point of stress about needing to get stuff done. Most times, I would end up throwing myself into a reactionary state and trying to cram activity into what was left of the late afternoon. And I'd almost always fail at getting in a good workout.

Starting the day early and getting out of the house as early as possible really does *set the tone* of the day. Even on days when I can work from home, I now make a point of waking up early and leaving my home for any reason possible because it gives me a jolt of energy and focus for my day.

> **RULE:**
>
> Wake up early and get out of the house!

Now that you're up early, what's next? How about breakfast?

Whether you like it or not, we all have to eat breakfast. Breakfast literally means "break the fast!" When you wake up in the morning after five to nine hours of sleep, you've been fasting—meaning, not eating for (hopefully) nine hours. Regardless of when you wake up, the first thing you eat, whether it's at 6 a.m. or 2 p.m., is technically breakfast—so we all eat it. *What time* we eat breakfast and *what we choose* is another matter, and that's what I'm going to talk about in this chapter. Let's go over the rules for breakfast.

Breakfast should be eaten *within the first hour of waking.* This is my rule, but I didn't make it up. This rule comes from a lot of research and personal experience. I've met many people who have reasons for not needing to eat early, but remember: This is *my* book, so you're getting my rules. Eat within the first hour of your day.

Here's my reason why: When you wake up in the morning, it's like turning on a gigantic power plant. Being asleep doesn't require much power, but getting out of bed requires a lot! Within about an hour after waking, assuming you're not eating a lot of sugar and pasta right before bed, you're probably getting to the point where you're getting low on blood sugar. Just by showering, brushing your teeth, and rushing around in your morning habits, you're burning sugar in the power plant that is your body. As soon as your innate intelligence detects that your sugar may be getting low, there is a "crisis" to deal with.

Your brain eats one thing and one thing only: glucose (sugar). If your innate intelligence gets the sense that your blood sugar is low, then it gets concerned that you will not be able to feed your brain, which requires a steady stream of glucose. So what happens? Well, if you don't get your blood sugar back up by eating, then your body's first reaction is to eat your muscles. Yes, your muscles—not the result you want if you want to be healthy. It would be great if it went after your fat stores first, but that just doesn't happen.

At first, you literally eat yourself through a process called *sarcopenia* (muscle breakdown), and after you've used your stored sugar from your muscles, your body can access another source of sugar from your liver through a process called *gluconeogenesis*. After those stores of sugar are used up (usually after about an hour or two) then and only then do you finally start to burn fat. The reason your body doesn't *only* eat fat is because it needs fat to survive, so it retains a certain amount of fat. Have you ever seen the show *Survivor?* They all lose weight because of calorie restriction, but they don't all get ripped beach bodies. Simply starving yourself causes you to lose muscle, so in order for you to truly be healthy, you must eat to support your muscle tone.

It's best to eat some sort of breakfast within the first hour of waking.

What to Eat for Breakfast:

Eat real food! Here are some good suggestions:

- A serving of nuts and seeds. Not a big handful—I would say about half a handful. The best ones are walnuts, almonds, pumpkin seeds, and chia seeds. Cashews are okay, too.
- A serving of fruit—organic is best!
- Eggs! So many ways to eat eggs!
- A serving of plain oatmeal, as long as it is not "Maple and Brown Sugar" flavored with all that added sugar. If needed, you can add a bit of maple syrup, agave nectar, or some bananas or berries, but not too much. You'll soon learn why—keep reading!
- Plain yogurt. Most flavored yogurts are no better than ice cream thanks to the added sugars and artificial sweeteners. If you need to make it sweeter, add your own flavor, as with the oatmeal.
- For all the grain-free paleo followers: Try two carrots, some slices of turkey, or even a piece of grilled chicken.

There you have it! Breakfast!

There are ten million other choices, of course, but I'm not going to tell you exactly what to eat every day. You need to understand the principles of how to choose wisely and why you need to choose wisely *yourself*, or you will never really change. Again, consult a nutritionist to find out what the best diet is for you, and make sure you're making healthy food choices, especially when it comes to your first meal of the day.

What Not to Eat for Breakfast:

- Processed foods: most things that come in a box with more than five ingredients
- Sugary cereals: If it has a cartoon character on it, just throw it out now!
- Anything made with white flour: At the very least, use whole wheat.
- Most flavored yogurts
- Cake: like Cinnabon! Bear claws, Pop-Tarts, most muffins, Danishes... . I know people eat these for breakfast, but they're really just cake.
- Can you picture the difference between food and junk now?

> **RULE:**
>
> Eat breakfast within the first hour of waking up! Start your day with food, not junk.

Set the Tone for the Day

"Set the Tone" is the name my friend and fellow chiropractor, Dr. Craig Fishel, gave to the morning conference call he used to host. The call was available for anyone to hear but was originally designed for chiropractors. It happened every morning, Monday through Friday, at 7 a.m., and its purpose was to literally set the tone for the day. It consists of a group-guided meditation and a breathing exercise that ingrains positive affirmations in your mind on the way to work. Check out the **49 Breaths** exercise later in this book for more details. Just think of how your day would improve if you heard like-minded people sharing a positive message with you every morning before work. I have found many other tools, audios, and books to listen to over the years. I make sure that I listen to something inspirational or uplifting every morning on my way to work.

Have a morning ritual that sets you up powerfully for the rest of your day. Recall that in Chapter 6 I talked about how to create a ritual—rituals are really just a collection of habits performed in sequence. A ritual is like a routine. You want to create a morning ritual so you can move through the same set of habits daily, setting yourself up for the day with a positive mindset. Here's my morning routine as an example that you can draw from.

Sample Morning Ritual

ALARM

My alarm clock is set for 4:45 a.m., but 80 percent of the time I don't need it—I am usually awake a few minutes before it goes off. As soon as my eyes open, my first conscious thoughts go toward prayer.

PRAYER

I was in a pretty bad car accident in 1995—ejected out of a car going sixty-five miles an hour and into the left lane of Route 80 in New Jersey. I was broken. In summation, I tumbled down the highway, resulting in road rash and cuts.

I separated my left shoulder, fractured my left collarbone, and had two compression fractures in my spine. During the ambulance ride to the hospital, I made a pact with God.... Isn't that always when we make pacts with God? When our lives are on the line? Well, in this pact, I decided that if I pulled through, I was going to do a lot of things, but at the barest minimum, I would recite the SH'MA every day (a Hebrew prayer basically praising God and thanking him for blessing me with another day). Ever since then, I wake up and recite the SH'MA prayer immediately. More importantly, on most days, I really mean it. I am thankful!

This accident was one of the major turning points in my life. I learned so much from it. Surviving a horrible trauma not only allowed me to appreciate life but also taught me what being a patient is like. Up until that point, I thought I had learned what it was like to be a doctor. After spending time on the other side, as a seriously injured patient, I saw the world through a different set of eyes. Eyes that now help me to understand healthcare from the patient's point of view.

GRATITUDE

After morning prayer, I get myself out of bed and use the bathroom. I then sit down on the edge of my bathtub, and I read my goals. I do this twice a day every day, as recommended and discussed in the amazing book *Think and Grow Rich* by Napoleon Hill—a must read!

I then turn on the shower and write down what I'm grateful for while I wait for my shower water to heat up. This is one of my favorite parts of my morning routine. When I'm writing my gratitude list, sometimes I put down big things, like something that happened recently that I'm excited about—for example, *Completing the manuscript of my life's work so I can express my passion for helping people improve their quality of life.* Or sometimes I write down the little things in everyday life that we take for granted, like, *The sun is out today.* Or, *I woke up today with a roof over my head and my family who I love safe at home with me.* (These "little things" are also big things, by the way!) Some days, the things I'm grateful for immediately jump out at me. Other days, I have to think a little bit about it. The benefit is that when I'm finished writing down what I'm grateful for, it puts me in a happy state that I take with me through the rest of my day.

Push yourself to write down three to seven things you're grateful for every morning.

GETTING READY AND BREAKFAST

Then I shower and start the day! After getting ready, I have breakfast. Remember, do this within your first hour of waking! Then I meditate!

MEDITATION

I cannot emphasize enough the power of meditation; in Chapter 17, I will cover meditation more in-depth, as well as provide explanations of different techniques you can use.

Finally, I'm off to the car for work!

COMMUTE

During my hour-plus commute, I always listen to something uplifting, whether it's a positive book, a podcast, or an interview with someone or something I'm interested in learning more about. Lately, I've been listening to Sean Croxton (**seancroxton.com**). No matter what, I must put something positive in my head before I get into the office. Listen to somebody talk about health or someone who inspires you or lifts you up. It doesn't matter who it is, but you should listen to something in the morning that puts ɔmething good in your head. As a result, time in the car that would otherwise be wasted can be implemented to improve your *Connectedness* and/or *Health Awareness* grades on the PRC.

When you visualize and plan your day, and when you begin the day with gratitude and positive messages, you will always have a better day because of it. The universe functions on laws of attraction. Like attracts like, so if you are placing positive messages in your brain on a daily basis before all of the "reality" of the day hits, you'll begin to shape *your reality* into what you envision. How do you start your day? Do you turn on the news? Do you immediately read your e-mails? *Stop it!* The news and the e-mails can wait.... . There typically isn't anything there that lifts you up!

The reason *Set the Tone for the Day* is one of the rules is because I don't want you to wait for a crisis before you take positive steps to change your life. I'll say more about the importance of feeding your mind with positive messages a little later, in Chapter 17.

All of these pieces of my morning ritual were developed over time, *not* overnight! I also had resistance to change. I'd hired a coach to help me improve my habits and rules and to hold me accountable to the routines I had created. When I was creating my ritual, I fought my coach on almost every suggestion he made. But over many months, I gradually did a little bit because I ultimately knew it was the right choice to implement these rituals, and, to be honest, I didn't want to waste all the money I was spending on coaching.

A great reason to have a coach: It keeps you accountable. During follow-up conversations, he praised me for what I had done and then asked me to do more. Each time I added a piece, my life improved. I don't know why we can't just snap our fingers and change; it really *is* that easy, but it seems to take a while. Don't worry, you have a lifetime!

Start with one change in your morning ritual at a time, and gradually add more until you're setting the tone you want for the day.

As you create your rituals, write down each step and keep it beside your bed or stick it on your bathroom mirror so you're always reminded of it first thing in the morning. Here's an example of what your morning ritual could look like:

> **Morning at a Glance**
> • Alarm
> • Prayer
> • Meditate
> • Gratitude/Goals
> • Shower/Get Ready
> • Breakfast
> • Commute/Uplifting Messages in Car

Going through each of the pieces of your morning routine—writing down things that you're grateful for every single morning, practicing meditation and mindfulness, and listening to something positive on your way to work—is an incredibly powerful way to set the tone for a great day.

Once you've created your morning routine, you can add routines to every part of your day. For example, I exercise most days (it doesn't have to be in the morning). And I journal at night before bed. Creating routines is a great way to implement new habits that will get you closer and closer to your goals.

Routines are important for keeping us on the right track and helping us establish new habits, but don't get worried about it not being perfect. Our lives aren't supposed to be perfect. Humans were put on this to survive, but for some people, that's all they do. Survive. They spend their time

.ng about chronic aches and pains. They're not living
: lives the truly want to live, and they're certainly not
.ving up to their potential.

We have this image from the media or something that
our lives are supposed to be amazing and perfect. For example, some preachers and motivational speakers make it
sound like everybody is supposed to have these amazing
breakthroughs every day—that we've been "chosen," and
today's the day. Even though I love these speakers and I appreciate the sentiment they're sharing, I also think it can be
a turn-off to some people.

If you're motivated by listening to people like Anthony
Robbins and Joel Osteen, but after a while you lose your
drive or feel frustrated that *today wasn't your day*, don't get
discouraged. You can keep on listening to these fantastic
motivators and spiritual leaders, as long as you also understand that you shouldn't feel frustrated if you haven't experienced the results yet. A mindset of success, health, and
abundance is a way of life... . Find your muse to keep you
focused along your journey. Also, remember that there are
plenty of muses, gurus, and teachers out there, so don't be
afraid to experiment with different ones.

By the way, I am one of those people who gets inspired
by people like Anthony Robbins and Joel Osteen. I can get
turned on and uplifted by the teachings of Buddhism and
Taoism as well. Keep learning and reading, and you'll find
what works for you.

Also, keep this in mind... . Nothing bad will happen if
you don't follow your routine perfectly every day. Remember, it's all about adding in more good. Don't focus on the
bad. Celebrate every time you do something in the routine
you've created. Just doing one thing a day from your morning routine will change your life. Remember to not be so

hard on yourself. This book isn't about being perfect—it's about getting *better*.

Okay. Now, you have my rules for making positive changes and my rules for setting yourself up for a successful day. These rules are a foundation that will enable you to make progress in each of the areas of your PRC. Now, let's dig deeper into each of the areas so you can see exactly how to bring up your grades. Use the rules we've talked about so far as the foundation for improving your quality of life in each area. If you find yourself struggling to make progress in any of the areas, come back to the rules in Part III and reread to review them. Making progress is simple, but it's not always easy. If you need to, return to Part III or write the rules from these chapters down and keep them somewhere visible as a reminder!

PART IV
Improving Your Grades on Your PRC

Now that you have your starting point, how do you go about raising your grades in each of the areas and your overall HPA (Health Point Average)?

In this section, I'll take you through how to raise your grades in each of the subjects on your report card. The following chapters are going to make a ton of suggestions/recommendations for improving your grades—remember the design of this book, and *take it one step at a time*! If you're working on improving one grade, then don't worry about the others yet! You may be a very high achiever who may try to improve all of your grades across the board all at once... And you know what? You may do it! But most people who try to implement too many changes at once eventually fail at them all because they get overwhelmed! Getting healthy is an ultra-marathon—*not* a fifty-yard dash. Take on whatever change you can handle and understand that if you're making your life even a *little* bit better, then you're winning the race.

Chapter 8

Diet

W e've all heard the saying "You are what you eat." This is very accurate. Simply stated, food is the essence of life. What we put into our bodies has the power to be life-sustaining or life-depleting. It's important that we know what to put in our bodies to make sure we give ourselves the best possible fuel.

I also want to tell you that I *love* food! I am passionate about food. I love to cook. I love to eat out at great restaurants. I will also tell you that I eat *whatever I want*! I want this for you as well! Life is short, and food is one of the greatest pleasures that we can enjoy.

Over the years of experimenting with my diet, I have learned which foods make me feel good and which ones don't. I used to enjoy eating all kinds of food, but over time, I limited my diet. I didn't feel deprived by limiting my choices. I felt better! Now, I eat completely differently than I did growing up because when you figure out what foods make you feel good and you learn to make them taste great, then I believe you've found a bit of heaven on earth!

Take a look at the grade you gave yourself in the area of *Diet*. Food and diet might be a challenge for you. It's possible that instead of being a source of nourishment, food has become an area of conflict and confusion for you. Are you enduring endless weight loss dramas, cravings, addictions, body image obsessions, and never-ending searches for "the best" nutritional system? Use this section to help you simplify food and diet. Keep in mind that the *rules* should be simple.

That doesn't mean that the implementation is simple. That simply depends on the rules that you create for yourself and how different they are from your current lifestyle.

I have had patients that have transformed their diet from a D to an A within weeks. I have seen others who have had immense struggles going from a B+ to an A because they just couldn't resist their one cheat food. I don't want you to be too hard on yourself during this process. Don't think of your diet as a thirty-day program. Your diet is simply the way you choose to eat. It is a lifelong habit, not a fad. And since it's a lifelong habit, it also means that you don't have to be perfect. In the upcoming pages, I am going to describe my rules. I will tell you right here and now though that *I do not follow my rules all the time.* My rules are the guidelines that I live by to make choices in my life. Over years of trial—and lots of errors—I have found out what works to keep me healthy.

The 80/20 Principle

I use the 80/20 principle in a slightly different way than it is used traditionally. Do a Google search if you want to learn more. Here is my version of the 80/20 principle and how to use it to help with your choices when it comes to your diet and how well you follow your rules.

Let's say that you've been following your rules for diet, but you totally screwed up one night and ate like a pig after a few drinks with friends. Okay, maybe you don't drink, but there are situations that come up where your willpower will be challenged, and you may break one of your rules. How do you deal with those situations? It all depends on whether you are in a time in your life when you want to make changes or you are in maintenance mode. Here is where the 80/20 rule comes into play.

- If you follow your rules 80 percent of the time, then I typically find that you maintain your current health status. You don't get any better or worse.
- If you follow your plan less than 80 percent of the time, then you are probably living a lifestyle that allows you to become less healthy over time.

    Additionally, if you are following your rules less than 60 percent of the time, then you don't really have any rules.
- If you are following your plan 85 percent of the time, you'll make slow changes.
- If you are following your plan over 90 percent of the time, your changes will happen more quickly.
- If you want to make a dramatic change, then simply follow 100 percent.... *No exceptions.*

Get the picture? Be honest with yourself. Create your rules and abide by them, but you can give yourself some slack if you are okay with making changes a little more slowly or if you are just in maintenance mode.

I'm going to talk about two things in the following section: *When* to eat and *what* to eat. Implement some of these rules, and in no time, you'll see your grades go up in this area!

First Basic Rule of Food!

J.E.R.F. Just Eat Real Food!

What does that mean? Simply think about what you are eating before you eat it. Ask yourself a simple question. Where did this come from? Ask yourself, "How many steps were taken in processing this thing I'm about to eat before it got into my mouth?" Examples:

Steak. Now I'm not talking about organic or grass-fed or how the animal was treated here. Those are questions I ask about my food as well. For now, I'm simply asking, "What had to be done to get this on my plate?" Is there more processing in a sausage? Yes. More ingredients were added. Let's take a can of sloppy joe mix. Was more processing done to that meat before it got onto your plate? How about that frozen dinner? Those chips? That cereal? The more ingredients on the label, the more processing was done. Does what you are eating look like it did on the farm? Did it take a completely different form?

Let's give some examples of minimally processed food, or food you would have to process yourself, meaning that you would have to cook it or prepare it in some way to make it taste good. Or not—maybe you could just eat it as is. Broccoli, chicken, egg, orange, fish, watermelon, squash, tomato, lettuce, bok choy, cauliflower, spinach... . Do you understand? If there is a single word that can describe all of the ingredients of the thing you are about to eat, then it's probably food. Then you can mix different foods together to create a multiple-ingredient meal—multiple ingredients that all started off as food—like a salad with grilled chicken. Not some frozen dinner with ingredients on the label that you can't pronounce.

The next thing to think about when it comes to J.E.R.F. is, does the thing that you are about to eat spoil easily? Ask yourself, "If I left this on the kitchen counter for a couple weeks, what would happen to it?" If it's highly processed, then it will look exactly the same as it did before. If it's *food*, then it will have at least started to spoil or rot.

Another simple question you can ask: "Is this going to nourish me?" If the answer is no, then it's probably going to harm you in at least some small way. You innately know that a donut is not nourishing and a salad is. You know the difference between junk food and something healthy, don't you? Well, if you choose to eat something nourishing, then your body will thank you, and if you choose otherwise, then your body will spank you!

Was this highly processed? Where did it come from? Will it spoil? Is this nourishing? Now that you know the questions to ask of the ingredients that make up your meal, start to make **better** choices! J.E.R.F.

How My Grade in Diet went from a D to an A

I want to give you some background on my quest for a healthy life and some of the first rules I created for myself.

I grew up as a very picky eater. I probably limited my diet to fifteen or so foods, and even then, I had rules for eating those. I loved tuna fish, but it had to be eaten on an English muffin—two different foods could not touch each other on the same plate. Ice cream *had* to be chocolate— plain chocolate with no chips. There are lots of picky kids out there (unfortunately, my oldest daughter inherited that trait from me).

Eventually, I freed myself from this prison of picky eating by the age of eighteen. How? I pledged a fraternity and while pledging, I was asked, expected, coerced, and forced to eat a lot of disgusting things; at least, as a picky eater, I thought they were gross! I can remember giant frozen sardines, head cheese, uncooked hot dogs, a giant can of cold Chef Boyardee ravioli, the hottest buffalo wings on the planet.... Why was I asked to do these things? I have no idea, but as a naïve freshman in college, I went along with the game. Afterward, I figured if I could eat this crap, I could try a slice of Swiss cheese, which I had despised until college. Thus, my rules for eating were broken.

This did not make me a healthy eater *at all*. Most of my life, I ate junk food if I had the choice. I used to have McDonald's hamburger-eating contests with my friends—five was my max—but I had no consequences most of my life. I could eat whatever I wanted, and I still remained a skinny kid. Physically, I felt okay, so why change? It was a life of pizza, hamburgers, General Tso's chicken, KFC, bagels, and ice cream.

Luckily, my mom was a good cook, so I did eat meatloaf and fried chicken cutlets a lot. I even liked peas and broccoli, so I wasn't exactly *ruined*, but by age twenty-six, everything began to change—I developed acid reflux. Even though I learned a lot about nutrition in chiropractic college, I never followed any rules about the quality of my food.

But when I began having symptoms—that changed it all.

The main lesson that I learned from becoming a chiropractor is that we all are born with an innate intelligence: the intelligence we were born with that keeps the body healthy and alive. If we're in touch with that innate intelligence and truly listen to it, it will *always* guide us to making the right decisions. I *knew* when I started developing symptoms that I needed to make a change in the way I was eating.

So what made me want to improve the quality of the foods I was eating and raise my *Diet* grade? The reason was not something vain like wanting to look better (of course, I *did* want to look better, but that never got me to make the right decisions about food). It was because my body was speaking to me. It was giving me a signal—a symptom: acid reflux.

Instead of looking for a pill or a quick fix to get rid of the symptom, or just dealing with it because it wasn't so bad, I asked myself *why*? *Why* was I getting this symptom? If you truly seek an understanding of *why* your innate intelligence has decided to give you signal or a symptom—acid reflux, anger, guilt, anxiety, irregular bowel movements, high blood pressure ... mostly anything—you will discover the answer. Then you can fix it!

And here's the most important part: If you *don't know why* it's happening, look for the answer in changing your *habits* or learning new *rules* for yourself before you jump to getting some drug or surgical procedure.

Your quality of life is the sum total of all of your rules and habits. Look there first. Make some changes and see what happens. *That's what healthy living is all about.*

> **RULE:**
>
> Listen to your innate intelligence about any symptoms you're having and look for the solution in changing your food rules and habits.

Eat Five Times a Day!

In Chapter 8, you learned the basics of breakfast. Remember to eat within the first hour of waking and simply eat food instead of junk! Here's a guideline for the rest of your day.

Again, this is a *guideline* to support you in making proper choices on your own. Everyone has different taste buds and different bodies, and you may find yourself in a situation where your preferred food isn't available. Sometimes, there are days when you can't have exactly what's perfect—you're stuck at an airport, you're at a conference in Omaha, or you're going to a friend's house for dinner, for example. I'll talk about what to do in specific situations like these a bit later. For now, here's your general guideline for what to do after breakfast.

The first part of this rule is: After breakfast, you *should* be hungry again within about three hours. The next part of the rule: *You should eat!* Now, repeat that three more times, and you'll be eating at least five times a day.

Why eat five times a day? I like to use the sumo wrestler/ bodybuilder analogy. Do you know how often the vast majority of bodybuilders eat? Well, it's anywhere from five to nine times a day—small, well-portioned meals that fuel their body's ability to build muscle. On the other hand, how often does a sumo wrestler eat? It's actually one to two times a day! The regimen I've read at a few sumo training facilities is this: Wake up, go to the dojo, do your sumo workout and learn skills for about four hours, then come home and prepare a *huge* meal, and *then* eat. Then, immediately after eating, they take a nap. They wake up after a couple of hours and go about their day as a sumo wrestler: cleaning up, hanging with their sumo bros, getting their bikini lines waxed ... whatever a sumo day consists of. Then they come home and prepare another *huge* meal late at night, eat, and go straight to bed.

Here's the point: Professional bodybuilders, over the course of many years, have figured out that the way to build muscle is to eat smaller, well-balanced meals many times a day. And over the many years of sumo research, they have learned that the best way to put on massive size (but not necessarily muscle) is to first stress the body by starving it, then feed it large amounts of food at a single sitting, and then rest or sleep.

Now think about *your* habits. Are your habits closer to a bodybuilder's or a sumo wrestler's? Let's work on getting them closer to a bodybuilder's habits. Eat your second meal within two to four hours of your first meal. Remember: Eat every three hours, on average.

Things can go wrong between two meals. What does *wrong* mean? Well, if you aren't hungry, I don't want you forcing yourself to eat. If you understand why you aren't hungry, you can prepare better next time. If you aren't hungry within three hours of your previous meal, there are three reasons why (four, if you count sleeping, but I don't):

1. YOU ATE TOO MUCH!

One of the reasons we aren't hungry within 3 hours of our last meal is simply because it was too much food. If we overeat we'll usually be full for a longer period of time. This may decrease the frequency of you meals. So if you aren't hungry 3-4 hours after a meal then ask yourself if you simply ate too much for one sitting?

2. YOU ATE TOO MUCH STARCH OR TOO MUCH OF THE WRONG FOODS FOR YOU!

If I have a bagel in the morning or a big bowl of oatmeal or the dreaded pancake (notice the word "cake" in there), then I feel bloated and full, and I probably don't need to eat for many hours afterward. If you're bloated after meals or after eating certain foods, you may *feel* satisfied and full, but you haven't satisfied your body's needs for proper nutrient intake. You may have had enough calories, but if the quality of the food you ate is low, the bloating may keep you from eating soon after. This is *not* the right way to become a bodybuilder! When should you bloat after a meal? *Never!*

3. YOU'RE JUST TOO DAMN BUSY!

If you don't think you ate too much, you didn't have any starch, and you don't feel bloated, a lack of hunger is most likely due to *stress*. Stress is a hunger suppressant. It doesn't have to be butterflies in your stomach stress but can merely be the stress of being busy. Think of it this way: 50,000 years ago, people woke up without any food. Each day, they had to hunt and gather or simply go without. If cavemen had been really hungry during their hunting/gathering, it would have been distracting, and they wouldn't have been able to work together to nab a wooly mammoth. If the mind is really busy, you aren't hungry (unless, of course, you're in a cooking class or something). If this is the reason you aren't hungry, then don't *force* yourself to eat; but you should *encourage* yourself to eat. Simply take a short break and get yourself in front of some food. See how fast your appetite turns around.

Being aware of those reasons should help you stay on track for eating frequently!

> **RULE:**
>
> Eat frequently—at least four times a day!

What to Eat for Lunch

This one is really easy! Do you want to know my rule for lunch? Eat a salad! That's it—just *eat a salad*! No, I don't care that you're in the mood for something else or that you had a salad yesterday ... and the day before that and the day before that and the day before that... . I don't care if you're bored with salads! Get over it and just have a salad!

Now, you can have a variety of ingredients *in* your salad—even different dressings every day—but you still need to have a fresh salad for lunch. Want to hear why I think it's a good idea?

- All of us need to eat more veggies!

- We need more fiber in our diets.
- We need more raw foods in our diets.
- We need more water in our foods—yes, salads are filled with water if you choose the right ingredients.
- They taste GREAT!
- There are virtually limitless combinations of ingredients so they can taste different every time.
- A salad carries a low calorie/high nutrient ratio.
- You can probably cram five to six servings of veggies in at one sitting.
- There will be fewer processed foods in your diet.
- It's just a good habit!
- Did I mention the low calories yet?
- And finally, *phytonutrients*!

Phytonutrients

I am purposely taking this opportunity to segue into the conversation about why we should be eating more vegetables and fruits, and also why organic is better. As I shared in the previous chapter, I eat a lot of nuts and vegetables, and I encourage you to do so, too, if you want to raise your *Diet* grade. Here's why.

Phytonutrients are the parts of plants that make each plant what it is. They are things like arabinogalactans, pycnogenol, sterols, stanols, carotenoids, ellagic acid, flavonoids, resveratrol, glucosinolates, phytoestrogens ... and the list goes on. I'm not here to give you a chemistry lesson, but I am going to give a quick summary of what these things are and why we should eat them.

These are the ingredients in plants that allow them to survive in nature, fend off mold and some insects, and make them taste a certain way. They have lots of different beneficial properties. The remarkable thing about this whole classification of natural food ingredients is that we have just scratched the surface in understanding what they do for us. The thing we *do* know is that the majority of edible plants that contain phytonutrients are beneficial. These nutrients support our immune systems, are great for our cardiovascular systems, calm our stress levels, and more. Sure, there are poisons, too, but we don't eat certain mushrooms because we know they're poisonous. The phytonutrients that are great for us are found in foods that we traditionally would consider edible sources of energy.

The best way to describe how phytonutrients work is by telling you the wild blueberry story. I heard this on an interview on Science Friday, a weekly radio show broadcasted on NPR. It's a great source of information—it basically highlights the top stories in science from the past week. Anytime I can plug into it, I will.

The story highlighted a certain species of wild blueberry that grows along the coast of Maine and up along the coast of Canada. For a blueberry to survive in such an unforgiving environment is a feat in and of itself: There's harsh sea air, extreme wind, cold temperatures, and rocky terrain.

Before I continue, let me first stress that blueberries are very good for you. Some of the phytonutrients they contain include ellagic acid, a phytochemical that has anti-cancer properties. It has proven helpful in the fight against breast cancer. Blueberries are also a good source of vitamin K, which plays a role in the prevention of liver and prostate cancer. They're also rich in antioxidants. Some of these, such as pterostilbene, help to reduce cholesterol in the bloodstream. Pterostilbene has also been established as an effective anti-diabetic agent. Other benefits of this antioxidant extend to supporting heart health, enhancing memory, and cancer prevention. The rich antioxidant content in blueberries gives them a high capacity to fight free radicals.

As for the super-blueberries growing in Maine and Canada, they have endured a harsh climate for thousands of years and have developed these ingredients to help them survive. So, if we eat these blueberries, they're good for us. Now, compare these resilient, tough but tasty blueberries to conventional blueberries that have been hand-picked for their size and taste, are grown in the best possible climate to maximize yield, have been sprayed with pesticides, and are given all the fertilizer and water they need for optimal growing conditions. There *is* a difference.

I am not saying that conventionally grown food is *bad*—we need it, too. Humanity has developed brilliant methods for cultivating food crops over the centuries. But they just don't compare to the wild. Sure, we need modern farming techniques to create volume, but very often, when you find a way to create more volume, you also lose quality somewhere. And since most of the food we are exposed to today comes from this massive-yield farming system, it's not as nutritious as the foods we used to eat.

- Now, I'm not suggesting that you go pick a wild salad of dandelion greens from the park. I just want to impress upon you the power that's inherent in natural foods. The life in your foods turns into the life in *you!*

- When you ask yourself what you're in the mood for, will you be basing your decision on peer pressure from your lunch mates or office mates, which is essentially relying on your stress levels to make your decision—and stressed-out people tend to pick bad foods—or will you start making some new choices? Break your old bad habits concerning food. Make the decision and *just stop it!*

- Before I conclude this section, I have to assume that there are some people out there who may want to try the salad rule but are concerned about missing their burgers and fries. Don't be discouraged. I promise you, a salad can be delicious. I look forward to my salad each day. Mine consists of one of my favorite combinations, but I play around with variations all the time, depending on my cravings. If you are new to eating salads, try choosing ingredients that you like from the list below.

SOME GREAT SALAD INGREDIENTS:

- Lettuce: mesclun mix, spinach, kale, cabbage, romaine—not just iceberg, please!
- Protein: grilled chicken, shrimp, hard-boiled egg, tuna
- Avocado
- Peppers
- Broccoli
- Beans
- Lentils
- Quinoa
- Carrots
- Squash
- Artichoke hearts
- Olives
- Tomato
- Beets
- Sunchoke
- A few raisins or craisins—not too many
- A few nuts or seeds—not too many
- Cauliflower
- Brussels sprouts
- Any sprouts

SOME APPROVED DRESSINGS:

Have any dressing you want—just watch it. The calories should never exceed 200. My suggestions:

- Lemon and olive oil
- Vinegar (balsamic or apple cider) and olive oil
- Vinegar alone

- Try changing your dressing each day, but don't use too much

My current salad of choice from Chopt, where I go for lunch, is:

- Kale, broccoli leaf, and purple cabbage base
- Avocado, black beans, chickpeas, squash, beets, broccoli and charred red onion.
- Balsamic vinaigrette dressing.

My wife Stacey's favorite blend is:

- Romaine lettuce base
- Avocado, grilled chicken, cucumbers, olives, broccoli and spicy peppers
- A little olive oil and hot sauce on top.
- This is a habit that is surprisingly easy to implement, and it will do wonders for your life!

RULE:

For lunch, *just have a freakin' salad!*

What to Eat for Dinner

Dinner should not be your biggest meal of the day. Recall the habits of the sumo wrestler versus the bodybuilder. Dinner should simply be another small portion—one of the five meals you eat each day. What you choose for dinner will depend on what the right diet is for you. Remember to consult a nutritionist for advice on choosing the right foods.

Let me give you my take on the best dinner. It's what I have for dinner about 90 percent of the time: a mix of protein and veggies—yes, more veggies! I get around seven to nine servings of vegetables a day (each serving equals one handful). Remember, if you increase the number of vegetables you eat every day, it doesn't leave room for all the junk! So here are a few common dinners for Mr. and Mrs. Piken:

- Paleo turkey meatloaf
- Paleo turkey meatballs
- Turkey burgers without bun
- Grilled salmon
- Grilled chicken
- Crab cakes (gluten free)
- Cod with puttanesca sauce

All of the above are accompanied by a side—which covers two-thirds of the plate—consisting of:

- Roasted broccoli or cauliflower
- Pureed cauliflower (like mashed potatoes made with cauliflower)
- Steamed peas
- Sweet potato fries
- Grilled zucchini
- Roasted okra
- And fifty other combinations of veggies dishes that I get from recipes, watching cooking shows, or just making them up... . I'm really good at cooking veggies and making them taste good!

RULE:

Don't have dinner be your biggest meal of the day. Find out what foods are best for *your* body and eat those foods in a portion comparable to your other meals of the day.

Snacks

So let's say you didn't eat enough at yur meal. Or you have a long commute. Or you were just stuck in a meeting for five hours and didn't have a chance to eat, so you need to grab something.

A QUICK LIST OF GRAB-AND-GO FOODS:

- Nuts and seeds
- Jerky: organic beef, chicken, or turkey
- Dried fruit—my favorite are prunes—but be careful that there isn't any added sugar, and be careful in general because dried fruit is naturally high in sugar; just a few pieces.
- Carrots or celery with or without hummus
- Try water or tea—sometimes quenching your thirst will take away your hunger
- Meal replacement bar

Just try to eat food and stay away from the garbage. You already know the difference!

Additional Food Rules

Next, I'll give you my daily food routine as an example for you to draw from. I'll also elaborate on some other general rules that I follow regarding food.

I'm sure many of you want to know, "What does Dr. Piken eat?" I don't eat the same exact thing every day, and I don't have the "perfect diet." I eat well, and, most importantly, *I've figured out what works for me.* My diet changes from time to time based on my health goals. Here's a snapshot of what it's like now:

1. Breakfast: nuts/seeds (usually cashews or pumpkin seeds) thirty minutes after I wake up

2. Eight to twelve oz of H2O every morning with my supplements
3. Coffee soon after
4. Some source of gluten-free fiber (currently Mary's Gone Crackers) a little while after
5. 10 a.m.(ish): Meal replacement shake (currently Ultra-InflamX from Metagenics)
6. 2 p.m.(ish): Lunch (salad)
7. Forty oz of H2O on my drive home from work
8. Dinner: some protein/veggie combination (last night: paleo turkey meatballs with roasted broccoli)
9. After-dinner snack: 85 percent chocolate (last night: Green & Blacks brand)

This is my routine. The only meal I tend to think much about is dinner. I eat things I like throughout the day, but I don't think about what I'm in the mood for; I eat based on what will give me a great quality of life. Most of my choices are already made. I make enough decisions every day—I need to cut thinking out of the process when it comes to the food I eat daily, so I've created a diet based on my rules. I know I want seven to nine servings of fruit/veggies (mostly veggies). I know I want thirty-five grams of fiber, minimum. I know I want to eat four to five times a day, and I know I want to eat clean, healthy protein sources from humanely raised animals whenever possible. When you know your rules for food, choosing what to eat becomes easy, and you don't even have to think about it.

Your rules will keep you on track. If you are getting a C grade in *Diet*, check your servings. For example: Are you getting seven to nine servings of vegetables? If not, that's one way to boost your grade. Look at your rules and see where you can tighten up your daily habits and choices.

Sure, I stray from my rules, but whenever I do, I just go right back to them. They work for me. As soon as I feel like they don't, I'll change them.

GET CONTROL OVER JUNK FOOD

I don't know about you, but I have a few weaknesses—one of those weaknesses is that if you put a bag of any type of cheese-flavored puffed junk food in front of me, I will finish the bag. I don't care how big the bag is; you will have to wrestle this bag away from me, or I will eat until it hurts and continue eating some more. I have a similar obsession with fried rice and most Asian noodle dishes. This is why I have rules! For me, first and most importantly, *no* cheese-flavored, puffed junk food in my house! That's it—I just *don't bring it into the house*. If it's not available, then I won't eat it. If you know you have weaknesses, stay away from them! Simply *don't buy* the foods you are prone to binge eat. Then you won't have to worry about the temptation later. For me, that rule has taken on multiple forms. First, it was *no partially hydrogenated oils* as an ingredient in my cheesy treats—they're highly processed fats that wreak havoc on your body. So first, I could only have the "healthier" crap in my house. That was a nice first step, but I still had too many big bags of junk filling up my belly.

The next rule I added was that I could only eat those snacks if they were made with *organic or non-GMO corn*—another hurdle meant to prevent me from putting so much garbage in my body (I'll say more about GMO foods below). But although these were good steps along the way, the best rule of all was to *just stop eating the junk food altogether*.

But let's say that you don't have complete control of your pantry because you live in a home with other people who have different rules, and some of your favorite potato chips happen to be in constant supply in your kitchen cabinet. Do you simply resist? Well, of course you do—or at least you should. *Just stop it*! Don't even start. You know if you eat one, you're sunk: 2,000 extra calories, extra fat, extra carbs—you want to *win* your game. Don't be a loser!

If I lived alone, I wouldn't buy some of the things I find in the kitchen cabinet. But I'm happy I don't live alone. I have an amazing wife, two amazing girls, and a couple of dogs, too. Sometimes, there are things in my house that I have a hard time resisting. So when I cheat with food, I have a rule to follow: Stand right in front of the cabinet you take the chips from and *eat them right there*. By doing this, I avoid the mindless munching while watching TV. If I sit on the couch and have a whole bag of chips next to me, there's a chance that the bag will be empty in fifteen to twenty minutes. I don't believe I have great willpower *all the time*, so I simply follow my rule when I want some potato chips. Since I've adopted this simple trick, I find that I stand there for a minute or two, have some chips, then put them back so I can sit down to relax and watch my show.

Do you have a rule that gets you to stop mindless munching? If not, try this one… . It works for me!

> **RULE:**
>
> Just stop eating junk food! And if you still find yourself tempted, create a rule that limits how much of it you eat.

Avoid Genetically Modified Food

Before we move on, I want to say a little bit about GMO food here. In this country, genetically modified corn is the norm, and you're almost certainly eating it unless you look at your labels and choose otherwise. Genetically modified food is a big topic.

As with the rest of this book, I am not going into a scientific argument about who is right and who is wrong when it comes to the genetic modification of food. I don't care that we have been modifying foods for thousands of years. For example, the cabbage family—which includes broccoli, Brussels sprouts, and cabbages that are red, green, and purple and have different shapes and sizes—has been heavily modified thanks to human impact. Some of these changes happened because we selected the traits we wanted and crossbred them with age-old agricultural techniques over literally thousands of years.

The modification I suggest that you avoid is the GMO of the past thirty to fifty years. If your genetic modification happens in a lab ... *not good*. If you like Brussels sprouts and they were created in Brussels a few hundred years ago, before we had fancy labs, then go ahead and eat them.

I understand that modern genetic modification has improved the supply of food in the world and may be beneficial in some respects because there are a *lot* of people to feed. But the regular use of these "Frankenfoods" has *not* been researched for decades upon decades—at least, not by anyone who isn't also directly involved in the production of GMOs and benefits from their increased sales. So my rule about GMOs is to simply learn more about them and to avoid them.

What do you do if you find that you're getting bloated every time you eat? What if you have food sensitivities? What if you have digestive issues or bowel movement issues? See the Special Circumstances section toward the end of this book, where I've included some information on the AI paleo diet to help you with these issues.

> **RULE:**
>
> Overall, when it comes to food, conventional is necessary, organic is better, and wild is best.

Chapter 9

Supplementation

Supplements provide our bodies with much-needed nutrition. But shouldn't we just eat food to get nutrition? Why do we need vitamins, supplements, or meal replacements?

Well, the truth is, we *don't* need them. We don't *need* much to survive in this world. That's one lesson I was taught growing up. A TV with a remote control? It's not necessary. Atari? I'd hear, "It's not necessary, Jason." Commodore 64? "Jason, you don't need that." Or, "Why do you need a car? We live in Queens. There are buses, and you can walk."

I can now appreciate the lesson I was taught growing up about needs vs. wants because it allows me to appreciate abundant living all the more. Of course, growing up with my needs met and my wants put on hold was a challenge at the time, but in the long run, people who learn to delay gratification have much better lives.

So, why vitamins? Because, as I teach people now, we don't have to merely *survive*. We live in America—we're freaking lucky. We can *thrive*! The innate intelligence of our bodies can take a Twinkie and turn it into fuel for producing energy and running our bodily functions. There are people who live by eating junk food every day, sometimes at every meal. Look at the members of the Rolling Stones—a lifetime of partying and touring the world is not the best lifestyle, but they still keep going! The truth is, our bodies can be fed absolute crap and take a lot of abuse and still simply survive. Some people can even thrive, no matter *what* they do to their bodies. They can party, eat what they want, drink what they want, and they still seem to thrive. But I must warn you, these are the rare exceptions to the rules of healthy living. As for the rest of us, we have to follow some rules if we want to thrive.

Vitamins—or supplements, as I like to call them—do just that; they supplement your life. If we were really eating all the nutrients we needed in order to thrive in our diet, there would be no need for supplements. But who's doing that? Barely anyone. I've been practicing for over twenty years now. I have met only a handful of people who eat better than I do, and I know I don't eat perfectly. (I do a pretty good job, though!)

If you are a member of the small percentage of people who *do* eat the seven to nine servings of fruits and veggies, the right amount of grass-fed organic meats, nuts and seeds, and fish and cooks all their own food in order to get all of the nutrients that we require to thrive, then great! Maybe you don't need a vitamin or supplement. But wait—are you eating all organic? Does the "organic" label on your food mean that it is *100 percent* organic? Or was there a meeting one night in some government office where a "deal" was made with top food industry lobbyists that allowed an organic stamp to be placed on food that is *mostly* organic. Is your organic farm a few miles down the road from a gigantic factory farm that raises pigs and contaminates the water supply?

Because you can never be 100 percent sure about the quality of your food, I generally recommend that everybody take a good multivitamin. For the majority of people, I recommend a fish oil and a probiotic as well, and then a specialty supplement, depending on what they need. If you're already taking supplements, then when it comes to this part of your report card, you can start by giving yourself a grade on consistency. If you're not taking supplements at all right now, start adding some to your daily routine.

The point is, no matter how "good" you are with your diet, there is always some bit of nutrition that you don't get because farming techniques in this country have become all about quantity rather than *quality*. We *do* need supplements to support our diet. We need them to make up for the nutrients that are supposed to be in our foods but aren't. They are also needed so that we can compensate for the fact that we are all born with at least some genetic predispositions towards disease. We understand enough about the body these days to know that we can alter the expression of our "bad" genes by eating the right foods, taking the right supplements, and improving our overall lifestyle.

> **RULE:**
>
> Take supplements. We may not need them to survive, but we do need them to *thrive*. If you want to get the most out of life, just take them.

Of course, in order to do this, you have to know which ones to take. Here's my basic list:

- Multivitamin (a good one!)
- Fish oils (for most of us—not all)
- Probiotics (again, for most of us)

What does "a good one" mean when referring to a multivitamin? Why fish oils and probiotics for "most of us"? Only a health professional trained in nutrition and the benefits and risks of supplements can truly advise you. There are thousands upon thousands of websites, newsletters, infomercials, and advertisements that make thousands upon thousands of recommendations for which supplement is the "*best*" for you. There is very little chance that the average person or even the above-average person has enough time to understand all the ins and outs of the supplement industry. Should you trust the person behind the counter at your local vitamin store? Should you trust the recommendation of your friend because she "loves her new herb"?

The supplement industry is just that: an *industry* that is filled with people trying to make a lot of money with the "new and best thing." I've been studying diet and nutrition for twenty-five years full-time, and I definitely don't know everything. I do know enough, though, to make sure that what I prescribe to my patients is the best recommendation based on what I understand about them as a whole person.

My number one suggestion for finding someone who understands nutrition from a holistic perspective is to look for a nutritionist like myself, an applied kinesiologist, a chiropractor, an acupuncturist, a naturopath, or a functional medicine practitioner who has been prescribing supplements for years. I'll talk more about applied kinesiology in Chapter 15. When consulting a professional, do your homework! No one understands nutrition better than someone who's been personally using it to heal for years.

If you can't consult a health professional, then my best suggestion is to improve your grade in *Health Awareness.* What does that mean? Do some homework! Read articles about nutrition, find the website of a health practitioner who seems to resonate with you and take their advice. Make sure you get your information from multiple sources, though. If many sources are giving similar advice, you have a better chance of finding the truth. So what should you watch out for? Advertorials: advertisements disguised as news and advice. They are everywhere now. There are many websites and magazines and newspaper articles written under the guise of education but with the main goal of selling a product. That doesn't mean that the information is false; you simply have to verify it somewhere else.

To be honest, it's even challenging for me. I've read articles that quote scientific studies, and I hunt down the original study only to find that it's of poor quality. Just because a study was done on a supplement, positive or negative, it doesn't tell you the whole story. There are many "news" stories I have seen and read that discredit supplements, and most of those are reports that quote biased studies. Understand that media outlets have to make money, so the stories that get produced often have some financial agenda behind them. Thousands of studies have been conducted over the course of decades showing many benefits from a plethora of supplements, but you seldom hear about them.

What gets big publicity are the rare negative studies, though. I believe that this is because the media is in part financed by pharmaceutical companies. Pharmaceutical companies produce drugs; supplements compete with drugs... . You do the math here. This is why I state, again: You need to spend time learning for yourself, or you need to find a practitioner you trust to help you. Check out some of the resources at the end of the book to learn more.

Dr. Piken's Medicine and Supplement Cabinet

I thought I would list here the supplements I have at home and take regularly. This is simply a window into what I personally take. This shouldn't translate to your own list. I often have people tell me that they are taking "so many supplements" and they don't want any more. I remind them that all they have to do, then, is have perfect habits, great genes, and live in the country, not the city ... or simply live without thriving. These are in no particular order.

Recall that not every supplement is created equal. I didn't even touch upon the quality differences present in supplements. This book is a primer. Please take my advice and work with a pro! I change the supplements I take based on my health needs and any new information I learn. This is my current regimen at the time of writing this book.

- *Multivitamin:* something to cover the bases. I use Metagenics Phytomulti right now for myself, and my kids take chewable Catalyn by Standard Process. I also recommend ClearVite from Apex for a powdered supplement form.
- *Fish Oil:* two to three grams a day. I use Metagenics for my fish oils as well.
- *Probiotics:* I have three different types in my refrigerator and choose different ones at different times. I use a mix of the Metagenics line of probiotics and the Apex energetics line.
- *Turmeric:* I use Tumero from Apex. It's a tasty liquid, and it's combined with medium-chain triglyceride oil, which is important because turmeric is so much better absorbed if it's taken with some healthy fat.
- *Glysen-Synergy:* This is another product from Apex. I struggle with blood sugar stresses because of my family history—and from eating like crap for the first twenty-six years of my life. I pay the price now by having to take supplements to support blood sugar balance. As long as my diet is good and I take these supplements, my blood sugar levels are perfect.
- *Vitamin C, and extra B vitamins:* I use these because of stage two adrenal fatigue that I am getting better at controlling.
- *Estrofactors from Metagenics:* This one is my wife Stacey's. Since she started regularly taking this one, we've been blessed with less emotionally strenuous menstrual cycles. Yes, I take it sometimes as well; it supports the body's ability to detoxify certain chemicals

(xenoestrogens) in our environment that have an estrogen effect. So, in turn, it can support testosterone production.

- *Magnesium Glycinate from Metagenics:* also Stacey's. When taking this one regularly, she has an easier time with elimination. I take it occasionally to help with muscle relaxation.

- *Vitamin D:* I take 3,000 IU per day. I currently take Metagenics liquid D3. I get my Vitamin D levels checked at least twice per year to determine my dosage needs. More about Vitamin D in the following pages... .

- *GABA Support:* I use three different types; I vary the types because I only use these supplements when I'm feeling anxious or stressed and my mind is racing. At different times over the years, I have had different levels of stress—or what I call adgeda—and I use different blends depending on the severity of the symptoms. When I take nutrients that support GABA pathways (GABA is a neurotransmitter that helps provide a feeling of calm) I have less adgeda! My wife sleeps like a baby since she started taking it. GABA itself is a waste to take since it shouldn't cross the blood-brain barrier; if you take pure GABA and feel calm, there's a good likelihood that you have a leaky brain, which is a condition similar to leaky gut. Basically, it means that things that shouldn't be crossing the blood-brain barrier are. The supplements that I take support natural GABA production within the body. The three blends I use are Trancor from Metagenics and GabaCore and Gabatone from Apex. Of all of the supplements I've mentioned, these are the only ones that *must be taken with the supervision of a health practitioner.* The use of supplements that can possibly affect the way your brain functions isn't something you should play with.

Remember, this is *my* cabinet—find out what's best for *you*.

- *Nazanol* from Metagenics—Runny, stuffy nose? Too much mucous? I've been using this one for years as needed.
- *UltraInflam-X* from Metagenics—I've been taking this product for about fourteen years. It's a meal replacement shake that serves as a multivitamin-amino acid replenishment pre/post workouts and provides general anti-inflammatory support and L-glutamine to support gut health.

*Please remember that I am Not recommending that you take what I take. Decisions regarding your health and well-being should be discussed between you and your doctor. The statements regarding supplements here have not been evaluated by the FDA and are not a substitution for advice from your doctor.

Again, I switch up my routine based on my needs and based on new insights and scientific discoveries. I'm not a fan of people who don't understand physiology or the holistic way of looking at the body prescribing their own supplements or medications. Please find a great local applied kinesiologist, chiropractor, nutritionist, or functional medicine practitioner who can help you figure out what's best for you.

Other Ways to Get Vitamins: the Sun and Vitamin D

Out of all the chapters in this entire book, I anticipate being ripped apart, bashed, shamed, or ridiculed the most for this one. Remember, I'm not here to list studies and give you stats here. I just want to state what I have learned and believe, and I want to point you to some resources for more info. I also encourage that you have more conversations with your own health practitioner.

I'm sure there are plenty of dermatologists out there who won't agree with my views, but here's what I think: *The sun is not evil!* Sure, it is for some people; if you have a genetic predisposition or a personal history of skin cancer, then use protection. But I believe that we are way too sun-averse.

There is a receptor for vitamin D on every single cell in our bodies. That is our body's design, so that fact implies that vitamin D is essential for the optimal health of our bodies. The single best way to get vitamin D is by being exposed to the sun. Now, you don't really need *that* much exposure; I'm not telling you to walk around with a deep bronze tan or to get a burn (definitely don't burn), but allow yourself some time in the sun on a nice day and don't worry about sunscreen constantly. It's incredible how few people I check for vitamin D have optimal levels. Satisfactory is a score of 30 on your blood test, but the optimal level is between 50 and 80. You will be doing yourself more good than harm if you allow enough sun exposure to get your D up. If it's low and you are one of those people who shouldn't be in the sun because of your fair skin or because of a higher risk of skin cancer, then you really should be taking a vitamin D supplement.

How much vitamin D should you get? Get the amount that will raise your blood levels of 25-Hydroxyvitamin D (25OHD) to 50 to 80 ng/mL. You should check your levels every twelve weeks while determining the correct dose and one to two times a year to check for increased/decreased needs. The best time to check is in the middle of winter and in the middle of summer. Your needs will change, and everyone's needs differ, so the best thing to do is test your levels regularly.

For more information on Vitamin D, check out www. vitamindcouncil.org.

> **RULE:**
>
> Learn what supplements are right for you.
> Consult a healthcare professional for guidance
> or hit the books and start learning.

You now have my rules for how to improve your grades in *Diet* and *Supplementation*. Next, let's talk about how to bring up your mark in *Exercise* for a better quality of life!

Chapter 10

Exercise

Exercise is one of the most researched and written about health-related topics, and there is an overabundance of opinions on how, why, where, and what kinds of exercise are best.

I am about to summarize the entire world of exercise in a few paragraphs. Are you ready?! I'll start off with the rule this time. It's *very* simple.

> **RULE:**
>
> *Exercise!* It is not an option! In some way, shape, or form, on a very regular basis, you *must* Exercise if you want to be healthy!

Yes, you must exercise if you want to be healthy, plain and simple! As I have stated before, everyone's grade and report card will be different. As you grade yourself in *Exercise*, keep your life in perspective. Sure, an A might be doing an Ironman competition and an F might be a couch potato, but what does an A look like for *you*? If you take a dance class once a week and really enjoy it, along with walking the dog daily, then that's your A. Keep this in mind as we go: The most important thing is that your rules are right *for you.* As you get healthier and learn more, you may decide that the habits you thought were an A are really a B. With your newfound knowledge, you can reassess your grade and your new plan of action.

In this chapter we'll go over some general basics of exercise, including time and intensity, what's too little, what's too much, and the importance of doing what you love (or at least, what you can tolerate). Most of all, you'll see that showing up is the most important part!

Another point to understand when it comes to exercise is that you should NOT exercise to lose weight. Losing weight, improving your body composition, is mostly dependent on your diet. Like I stated before, exercise is a vital part of being healthy, but exercise will have a minimal impact on your weight loss goals unless you are spending many effective hours a day in the gym. So many people have come to my office over the years complaining that they can't lose weight. Some of these people are going to two spin classes and two boot camp classes a week on top of running two miles twice a week. They are putting all this effort into exercise, but then they're going home and feeling that they "earned" the right to eat whatever they want because of the hard work they put in. That just doesn't work. Please continue to exercise, but work on getting an A in *Diet* if your goal is weight loss.

When it comes to exercise, you need to understand a simple formula, the formula of time and intensity. It's very straightforward: If you don't want to spend a lot of time exercising, then you must make it intense exercise; whereas, if you don't like intense exercise, then you must spend a lot of time exercising! That's it. It's not too hard, is it?

Next, let's address these intensity levels. The goal should be to add enough exercise to your life to bring up your grade in *Exercise* without negatively impacting your grades in other sections. Play with that balance and find the right amount of exercise for you. You'll also want to start doing workouts you *actually enjoy.* If you like jogging outside, do more of that. If you enjoy following online exercise programs, do those. You're more likely to follow through on the rules you set for yourself if they involve something that also makes you happy.

Now ... just because I'm in a great mood, I'll give you a few more tips regarding exercise. Here's how to set up your exercise routine: First, pick the amount of days per week that you will exercise. Not how many days a week you think you *should* be exercising. Pick the number of days per week that, right now, starting today, you truly *promise* yourself you *will* exercise. Be honest with yourself—it doesn't matter if it's only one day as long, as you create your rule and stick to it. But also know that if it's only one or two days right now, then pretty soon it must become three. One or two days may keep you from turning into a big blob of goo on the couch, but you need at least three days a week to start to make changes in your body.

Okay. Now that you've determined the number of days a week that you're going to exercise, the next question is, how long are you going to exercise each day? Again, be honest and pick a number that works for you, even when your life is busy and crazy—don't promise two hours, three times week if you can only do forty-five minutes. And don't promise forty-five minutes when, in reality, you can only do fifteen. If, after you hit your rule minimum, you then decide that you want to do more, that's great. Just don't let yourself down by promising too much too soon.

Now that you've got your number of days a week and the amount of time for each session, let's get in the next pick: What are you going to do? Base this (at first) on the amount of time per week that you have allotted for exercise. Remember the ratios: low time/high intensity, high time/ low intensity. For example, if you plan on walking for exercise, then you had better give yourself at least ten hours a week of walking. Most people I know don't have that kind of time, however, so if you have less than ten hours a week for exercise, you need to incorporate at least a bit of strength training or high-intensity exercise.

And if you don't know what to start with, just *show up and move.* Walk and jump around and dance a bit. Sure, it would be ideal to be an exercise expert, but you aren't yet, so just *start moving.* The most important thing is to get your body moving.

Once you're moving regularly, start taking steps to learn what you can do to exercise effectively. You don't need to hit the gym and pick up massive weights—and in most cases, I wouldn't want you doing the routines that you picked up in high school, either. Learn how to exercise properly so you don't waste your time. I can't tell you how many people work out at the gym, wasting time, energy, and money, when if they would just learn how to work out properly, they would get closer to the results they want with every workout.

Here are some ways you can learn how to exercise better:

Hire a Personal Trainer

This is the most expensive option, yes, but a well-trained personal trainer will not only get you the results you want; he or she will also teach you how to use your body properly to build and sculpt it while avoiding injury. The last thing you want is to hurt yourself just as you are getting into working out and fall off the wagon.

Take Classes

Don't want a trainer? Or maybe you can't afford one or just don't have time for one. No problem. Join a gym and find classes to take. This option is not as personalized, but a good gym vets their trainers and approves the classes they host. Classes are a great way to get motivated and learn how to exercise.

GET WORKOUT VIDEOS

You say you hate gyms? Okay, get some videos. You don't need a gym! Between the online availability of virtual trainers and the world of Tony Horton, P90X, and **Beachbody. com** videos, there is an abundance of videos out there that will help to get you off your butt and moving. Just be careful not to push yourself too hard. I have seen far too many injuries resulting from people doing high-intensity videos before they're well-trained and ready. Start with something that matches your pace. The video I like the most for beginners is *10 Minute Trainers by Tony Horton.* For those who are truly committed and have a little more strength and experience, P90X with Tony Horton is another great video program that will get you fast results. I also recommend looking up Tim Senesi Yoga and Fightmaster Yoga on YouTube, and my current favorite for bodyweight workouts is Brendan Meyers. Just search "Brendan Meyers abs" on YouTube. I add it to the end of my workouts.

No matter what your level of experience with exercise, please keep in mind that fast results aren't always what you are looking for. Repetition is the key. You need to exercise on a regular basis, *forever!* It doesn't matter how quickly you get your results. I coach people to take baby steps and make commitments to avoid blowing up after six to eight weeks of intense training that they can't stick with. You can always add more later!

If this all sounds like too much for you, go back to the basics and just *get moving.* Find an activity or a sport that you like—or even just one that you can tolerate—and start there. Just do it already! By the way, dancing is also a fantastic exercise! So is tai chi, especially for those of you who are elderly or injured. Remember: *Just move!*

Let me give you an example of an exercise regimen that I recently worked on for a patient, Beth. I think the best way to understand the process I used to design Beth's plan is to recreate the conversation we had.

"All right, Beth," I said. "So, you've told me that you know you have to work out but you're not sure what to do."

"Yes, Dr. Piken," said Beth. "Let me tell you my daily routine. First, I need to get myself and my two kids ready for school and get them on the bus. By that time, it's 8 a.m., and I need to leave for work. I can't exercise during the day. It's too busy at work. I get home around 6:30 p.m., and I need to get the kids fed, help them with their homework, and get them ready for the next day of school. Also, I need to eat something, and I need to spend a few hours winding down and watching some TV or else I'll go mad."

"Okay, Beth," I said. "That definitely is not the optimal schedule for a person who wants to introduce regular exercise into their routine, but let's give it a shot! What time do you wake up?"

"6:30 a.m."

"Okay. Can you wake up fifteen minutes earlier?"

"Yes, I can do that!"

"Okay. How many times a week do you really think you want to exercise?"

"I would really like four days a week."

"Can you exercise on the weekends?"

"Yes, I have a little more free time on the weekends."

"How does this sound?" I said. "Choose two weekdays, any weekdays, to wake up fifteen minutes earlier. I would recommend Tuesdays and Thursdays because I also want you working out on Saturdays and Sundays. Have your exercise clothes waiting right next to your bed so you don't have to waste any time getting dressed. Find a place to exercise. Then Google the words "10-minute intense exercise" and go to the video section. The last time I did this, I got 141,000 videos to choose from. Pick a video that has a description that matches your mood and *go!* You can pick a new video every day, or you can do the same video every day. If it feels too intense, Google "10-minute yoga" instead. The last time I Googled that one, I got 1,200,000 selections. On the weekends, when you have more time, how much time do you think you could promise yourself that you will use to exercise?"

"One hour," said Beth. "I can do an hour on Saturday and Sunday."

"Great," I said. "Do you like to hike? Play tennis? Swim? Jog? Kickbox? Do you get the picture? It's up to you to choose what you're going to do, but if you have an hour, try doing things you enjoy. And if you don't have enough time for those things, then get to those videos again and type in the time that you have.

"Now, to summarize: Your goal is to exercise four days a week for a minimum of fifteen minutes a day two times a week and one hour a day twice a week. That means that if you wake up on Thursday morning and you haven't exercised yet, then you cannot miss a day for four days straight. That's why I suggested that you plan your days for Tuesday and Thursday. That gives you some makeup days if your schedule gets tough. Also, if for some reason you can add another day, great—*bonus!* Does this sound like a plan that you could keep up for the next four months?"

Do you see how it works? I just picked one of those really tough schedules for this example, but there are thousands of combinations of routines that could also be used. I'll simply end with that old saying, "Where there's a will, there's a way."

I touched on this before, but I'll mention it again. Exercise is *not* what you want to improve your grade in if your main goal is to lose weight or lose fat and change your body composition. If that is your goal, focus most of your energy on changing your diet. 80 percent or more of the changes that people really desire for their bodies come from diet, not exercise.

Think of it this way. If you spend twenty to twenty-five minutes running two miles and you burn about two hundred calories, you can come home and eat those two hundred calories or more in about two minutes and completely wipe out your gains. Okay—it didn't really "wipe out" the benefits of exercise. You can't erase the fact that you did something good for yourself. My point is, there is a huge misconception out there. Despite the years of research, people are still amazed when I tell them that weight loss and body fat loss is primarily based on what you eat.

So, why should you exercise? In summary, it is simply essential. Exercise improves your mood, your intelligence, your looks, your confidence, your fitness, your cardiovascular system, your immune system.... it improves *everything* you do and everything you are. Sure, there is a *ton* more information about exercise available, but this is not a book about exercise—it's a book about creating rules for yourself so you get into the *habit* of exercise.

> **RULE:**
>
> Get moving! Use the ratio of time/intensity.
> Learn how to exercise better.

The Difference Between Fitness and Health

Here's a bit of advice I use to get people to be realistic about their bodies and the shape that they should be in. I like to think of my body as a "six-weeks body." What that means is, at any given time, I could spend six weeks working out and eating even better than I do now, and I would have my dream body.

Why don't I have my dream body right now? It's too hard! That's right, I said it—it's way too hard for me and most other people to obtain and maintain a perfect "beach body" all the time. Just because the fitness models, TV stars, airbrushed magazines, and maybe even your neighbor or business associate has that perfect beach body doesn't mean that you need one all the time. I do believe that people need to be healthy (as evidenced by the entire content of this book), but being healthy and looking like you have a model-quality body are not necessarily congruent. They can be, but they don't have to be.

You see, there is a difference between fitness and health. *Health* means that your body as a whole is functioning the best it can, all the time. It means that there is nothing interfering with the innate intelligence of your body and its ability to repair itself. *Fitness*, on the other hand, has to do with looks and the ability to perform or accomplish athletic tasks. I have seen many fit people who aren't healthy as well as many healthy people who aren't fit. I've seen people running the NYC marathon and finishing in a decent amount of time; meanwhile, their body fat percentage is above 30 percent and they're stressed out at work every day. I've seen people who have perfect bloodwork, a low percentage of body fat, great genetics, and great nutrition who can't do one pull-up.

The best combination, of course, is to have both. But that usually means that you are spending an awful lot of your time devoted to fitness and health. Even someone like myself—whose job is to be healthy and fit as an example to others—could do better, but I have to balance my fitness level with time with my family, dedication to my office, and, to be honest, the love of having some wine, bourbon, or tequila with a good meal a couple of times a week.

For some people, being fit and healthy at the same time comes easily. For most of us, it's at least a bit of a struggle, and for many more still, it's an arduous, uphill battle with a knapsack filled with cinderblocks on our backs. Sometimes, where we *want* to be is different from where we *should* be. My recommendation is to focus on being healthy, and know that you can always get to your preferred fitness body within six weeks. I'm happy with my six-weeks body. If you are currently in a state where it would take you at least six months or more to get that "perfect body," then you need to shift your priorities and habits to close the gap. You are probably in a state that's not as healthy as you could be with a little more effort.

> **RULE:**
>
> If it will take you more than six weeks to have the body of your dreams, then get to work!

There's something else that I think is important to mention about exercise: If you invest in workout equipment, make sure you're actually going to use it! To illustrate this point, I'll tell you a quick story. This is one of the anecdotes I often use with my patients when helping them decide whether or not to buy workout equipment.

MOM'S TREADMILL

My mom bought a treadmill!

Woo-hoo! Great! My mom was going to start working out! I was super happy about that. *Wrong.* **Within hours of getting the damn thing set up, the treadmill became a new place to hang her newly washed clothes to dry. She** *never* **used it as a treadmill.**

Think about whether or not you're ready to really use a workout product or service before you invest in it!

> **RULE:**
>
> Only buy workout equipment and services you will actually *use*.

Exercise Makes You Smile

My daughter Ryan just reminded me of something I tell her all the time. (Maybe one day all the brainwashing I do for my kids will pay off! At least I know she's listening, even if she barely exercises. We'll see what happens as she gets older.) Ryan reminded me to mention that when you exercise, you feel better.

It's true. Whenever you're in a bad mood, there is no better sure-fire way to feel better than to exercise. I don't care if you don't like to exercise or you don't feel like it in that moment. Just get up off your butt and do it! I guarantee you will be better off for doing it, and you will be glad you did.

> **RULE:**
>
> Exercise makes you *smile*! You're only one workout away from a good mood!

Chapter 11

Body
Composition

To understand how to improve your grade in *Body Composition*, you must first understand exactly what "body composition" means. Body composition is your percentage of fat compared to your percentage of muscle. What we want, of course, is a high percentage of muscle. As we age, we tend to lose muscle—actually three to eight percent of muscle mass for every year of life, on average, and even more after age sixty.

Unless we're working hard at maintaining or even gaining that muscle, we're going to tend to lose it. The decline starts after the age of thirty. If you haven't built your muscle by the time you're thirty years old, you had better start doing something right now, because you don't have those reserves built up. Muscle percentage is actually the number one biomarker of the aging process; it's the number one factor in determining how well you're going to do when you're older and how healthy you're going to be.

The best way to assess your current muscle percentage and body fat percentage is by going to a doctor or a personal trainer who is highly trained at measuring muscle. If you're going to do an estimate on your own, you can use the grading guidelines from section 1 and grade yourself based upon the flatness or tone of your belly. Keep in mind if you base it all on your belly area you may over/under estimate because of your body type. Also, you can estimate based on what you personally think of your body. Do you think you're in phenomenal shape or do you think you are in "okay" shape? This is a self-graded, subjective test. The important thing is that you should always be honest with yourself.

The important thing is that you should always be improving your body composition, no matter your starting point.

I'm going to give you a couple of examples from my own life to illustrate the importance of building up your muscle mass *now*. My grandfather, at the age of eighty, retired from being a glazier. A glazier is somebody who works with glass and windows. He worked hard, physically, his whole life in his profession. When he finally sold his shop and retired, I remember being with him in front of his store in Brooklyn. He said, "Jason, feel this." He was flexing a bicep really hard, and he said, "Feel it. Poke it." I did. It was rock-solid.

Being an eighty-year-old man with a rock-solid bicep is why my grandfather lived until ninety-nine years old and had very few to no physical problems until maybe the last year-and-a-half of his life.

Now, contrast this with his wife, who is still alive. Thank goodness I have my grandmother still around! She's about to turn ninety-two. In contrast to my grandfather, she never really physically challenged herself. She loved to walk. I'm going to break this to you gently, but walking is not exercise. Walking is great for your heart and your mental state. It makes you feel good mentally, is fantastic for your brain, and gets your heart pumping a bit, but unless you're really pushing yourself or walking many, many miles, it doesn't build a lot of muscle mass.

My grandmother liked to walk mainly for her brain, so she didn't walk fast. Because she didn't eat in the best way possible and she never really strained or physically worked her muscles, her body did degenerate over time, and her mind eventually did as well. She's doing okay for a ninety-two-year-old with dementia, but physically, she needs assistance getting around everywhere. She requires the use of a walker and needs to be pushed just to walk a little bit. Basically, because she was never really physically strong in terms of a high percentage of muscle, she has been stricken with a life of needing help—not only mentally but physically—just to get around and change her clothes.

I want something better for myself. I want something better for you, too. In my situation, I know my history. My family history indicates that there might be some mental challenges down the line. Dementia and mental faculty have a lot to do with blood sugar, which is one of the reasons I'm so diligent about what I eat and don't eat. What I really want to do is to beat my grandfather's record by being able to physically care for myself when I'm in my eighties and even into my nineties. As I mentioned right at the beginning of this book, I want to be able to cut my own toenails. I want to be able to play golf, play tennis, go hiking, walk my dogs, and play with my great-grandkids in my old age. I want to plan now in order to be able to do those things later. If you're not focusing on the percentage of muscle that you have—if you aren't constantly stimulating, growing, and challenging your muscles—then you're going to wind up either playing catch-up later or simply suffering.

Hopefully, these examples illustrate that your body composition is something you should pay attention to! The general rules are as follows: Males should be under 20 percent body fat; optimum is a little closer to the mid to low teens. Males definitely want their body fat under 25 percent, meaning 75 percent muscle or greater! Of course, as we get older, some natural loss is going to happen. It's a lot more difficult to have the same percentage of muscle in your seventies and eighties that you did in your twenties, but it *can* happen. I've seen people push themselves and make it happen.

For women, the optimum body composition is between 20 and 25 percent body fat. That's a wide range. This is because of different body shapes, plus the natural variations in the sizes of hips, breasts, and buttocks. When women hit menopause, the optimum body fat percentage gets closer to 30 percent, but you still want it to be under 30 percent. Of course, again, as you get older, you have to work harder at maintaining that. What this means is that you have to be tighter in your diet and make sure you're always stimulating your muscles.

There's a book called *Biomarkers* by William Evans, PhD and Irwin H. Rosenberg, M.D., in which these two researchers from Tufts University found ten modifiable markers that can be used to measure and impact physical decline with age. They found that the number one and number two factors in impacting the aging process were: *percentage of muscle* and *strength*. Of all ten markers, these two were the strongest in predicting how well one would age.

They also found that of all the markers, the one that had the most impact on all of the others was increasing the percentage of muscle. Therefore, if you can only pick one goal when it comes to having high a quality of life for the rest of your life, it should be to have a high percentage of muscle. As sarcopenia (the gradual loss of muscle during the aging process) occurs, which happens from about age thirty on, we technically start to lose our muscle mass every single year as part of a natural process—*unless we do something about it.*

So *how* do you do something about it? The two main ways to improve muscle mass are exercise and diet. While each was explained in detail in the previous sections, I'll add one more important thing in here about diet: If you want to build muscle and prevent muscle loss, the number one factor has to do with one simple ingredient: sugar.

When I say sugar, I don't just mean refined sugar; it's also alcohol, starchy foods like potatoes, rice, bread, and even fruit. The body's requirements for sugar are low—we don't need much. What happens if we have enough sugar in our body and we put in more than we need? A hormone called insulin gets released. What does insulin do? It says, "Well, we've got all this extra sugar. What the heck do we do with it?" It says, "Okay. Let's put it into these little packages right here." Those little packages are called fat cells.

The vast majority are putting in more sugar (refined sugar, alcohol, starch, and glucose) than we technically need. All that extra starch and sugar is being stored as fat. Remember, the number one thing we need is muscle, not fat. So technically, if you truly want muscle, lower the amount of starch you eat. Try getting rid of all starches for temporary periods of time (I wouldn't recommend cutting them out altogether forever), such as one or two days a week, three or four days a week, six months at a time, or two years at a time … whatever it takes. It will slow down muscle loss and sarcopenia.

Exercise also lowers blood sugar. Every single time you contract your muscles, you're helping your blood sugar. Keep working your body. Ultimately, if you stop working your body, it stops working for you. The important thing is to keep your body moving. If the body is not moving in some way, it is dying.

Here's the main thing to know about body composition: It's the result of how you're doing in all of the other areas of your report card. Your HPA (Health Point Average) reflects a summary of all your habits. Similarly, your body composition—your percentage of muscle and percentage of fat—is reliant on the combination of so many different factors. It's a result of the combination of how much water you drink, how much sleep and rest you're getting, how often you're exercising, whether or not you're eating the right things, etc. Your body composition is like a barometer to tell you how you're doing.

Your grade in *Body Composition* is one of the most important grades on your report card because it tells you how you're doing. It's like a feedback loop. Take your body composition seriously and use it to test how you're doing in the other areas. If you're over the target body fat percentage, make the appropriate changes in the areas of diet, sleep, exercise—and really, *all* of the areas on your report card—and see the changes in real time from one report card to the next. Measuring your body composition is a great motivator—as you see changes from one report card to the next, you'll know you're on the right track; and if you're not seeing changes, you'll know that you have to upgrade your grading scale or work harder at instilling new habits.

Now here's my favorite tool for measuring body composition. No, it's not a fancy scale that reads your body fat percentage. No, it's not the expensive DEXA study at an anti-aging clinic. It's probably something you already have in your closet at home.

So here's the story of Stacey, my wife, and the scale we used to have. My wife grew up learning many bad lessons about diet, weight, and body composition. She learned these, as many people do, from parents, friends in high school, trashy celebrity magazines, and, of course, *they*! As in, "You know what *they* say?"

For many years, Stacey thought the best way to assess her body composition was to step on a scale one to two times a day and stress about the numbers. I begged her for years to stop using the scale because there really is no ideal weight for anyone. It's all about the percentage of muscle you have and your shape, not your weight. I don't know about you as a reader of this book, but personally, I don't know many spouses/partners/couples that will listen to the advice of their significant other without a fight. This fight lasted about *ten years*! Until the miracle happened... . The fancy electronic scale finally ran out of batteries! She milked it for months, pushing on it, shaking it, saying "just one more reading!" But finally, I won! You see, I had made her promise that when the scale finally died, her habit of stepping on it over and over again would die as well, and she respectfully accepted the death of her scale as a sign that she needed to move on with better ways of measuring.

As a replacement for the dead scale, she needed something quick and easy and accurate. What did she choose? *The perfect pants*! Stacey had a pair of pants, a pair of shorts, and a pair of jeans that only fit right when she was at her ideal body composition. Her "new scale" turned into trying on one of these "perfect" items of clothing each day.

I accepted her "new scale" as a healthier alternative. It's great to feel good about how you look. It's a motivator to stay the course or to make changes. Of course, if it *isn't* a motivator but instead acts as a stressor, then don't use it! Use tools that motivate you instead of depressing you. For some of you reading this, the PRC alone can be your tool. If your habits are great, then you are great! For those of you who like numbers, go to a health practitioner who measures your body composition, or use the scales that measure body fat percentage (I just don't love their accuracy). Or maybe you like the Stacey method; try on your ideal pair of jeans or T-shirt or dress and see how it fits. Remember, the goal is *not* for ladies to be obsessed about fitting into a size zero dress or for guys to obsess over a thirty-inch waistline. The goal is to set a reasonable goal and work on it forever!

RULE:

Throw away your scale and work on your shape!

Chapter 12

Sleep

The most important sentence you read about sleep is this: *Sleep is the only time your body gets to heal.*

If you take in the information above, it should be enough information for you to pay attention your quantity and quality of sleep! These days, the average American is not getting enough sleep. In fact, insufficient sleep is now being treated as a public health concern. The Center for Disease Control and Prevention (CDC) considers insufficient sleep a public health problem in the United States. Data from the Behavioral Risk Factor Surveillance System (BRFSS) survey analysis indicated that, among 74,571 adult respondents in twelve states, 35.3 percent reported that they got less than seven hours of sleep a night, 37.9 percent reported that they had unintentionally fallen asleep during the day at least once in the prior month, and 4.7 percent reported that they had fallen asleep while driving at least once in the prior month. That's 3,505 people who fell asleep while driving—in a single month!

An excuse I often hear for lack of sleep is "I'm not tired." If you're truly not tired, that's great. But odds are, you might just not *feel* tired because you are so used to lack of sleep that you have gotten used to operating at a lower-than-optimal level. Also, just because you *can* do something without feeling the side effects doesn't mean that you *should* be doing it.

The human body is amazing; we can go without so many of the things that are beneficial to us ... including sleep. We can push our bodies and become accustomed to ridiculous life-styles. But just remember that every time you go against the rules and push your body, you're adding to the overall stress equation in your life. So here's my bottom line: Get your six to nine hours of sleep a night. I like seven and a half, myself.

Why is it so important to get enough sleep? The CDC notes that insufficient sleep has been linked to motor ve-hicle crashes, industrial disasters, and medical and other occupational errors.[2] Lack of quality sleep has been linked to every known neurodegenerative disease. It's been linked to anxiety, depression, Alzheimer's, dementia, and Parkin-son's Disease. Sleep disturbance is one of the earliest signs that the brain has been taking on too much and is likely to degenerate faster than people who *do* get great sleep.

Take sleep seriously; even if you think you've got enough energy during the day and think you don't need sleep, lack of sleep will catch up to you in some way. The CDC states that people who don't get enough sleep are also more likely to suffer from chronic diseases like hypertension, diabetes, depression, and obesity, have increased rates of mortality, and have reduced levels of productivity and quality of life.

Sleep deprivation has also been linked to poor perfor-mance. A recent study revealed that lack of sleep impacts people's ability to make decisions and adapt, especially in dynamic or changing environments. This finding has espe-cially important implications for people involved in careers like emergency response, disaster management, military operations, or other environments requiring fast response time. It was also found that getting longer periods of sleep improved athletic performance. A study conducted on eleven healthy male students on the Stanford University men's varsity basketball team found that with sleep exten-sion (longer periods of sleeping), the athletes' shooting ac-curacy improved, as did their reaction time, and they had higher overall ratings of physical and mental well-being during practices and games. The study further concluded that sleep is beneficial for athletes in reaching their peak performance.[3] Overall, it's been found that sleep deprivation affects levels of performance across a wide variety of physical and cognitive tasks.[4]

Sleep is incredibly important to our overall health, level of performance, and quality of life. But how do you make sure you're getting enough, consistently, and how do you know how much is enough? Furthermore, how do you make time for sleep with all of the other things on your plate?

Get Enough Sleep!

First of all, in terms of the rules about sleep, I don't think there is any magic number for the exact amount of hours of sleep that we really need. I know that sleep requirements are different for different people. That being said, I do have recommendations for rules that you can set up for yourself when it comes to sleep.

Although I don't believe there's a magic number of hours of sleep people should get, I do believe that there is a magic *range:* six to nine hours (as an adult). If you get less, you are compromising your ability to rest and heal. On the other hand, if you're sleeping more or feel like you *need* more than nine hours, then maybe there's something wrong with your overall health—either that, or we need to find you some passion or some drive to get out of bed earlier in the morning.

Sleep is awesome. Sleeping is one of our body's main, natural states of being. It's the time of peace and rest. Remember, it is the only time our body has a chance to heal, so if we are lacking sleep, then we are not allowing our body time for healing and recovery. It takes a lot of energy for your body to be awake and alert, which is technically stressful. You need stress hormones like cortisol to help you to function while you're awake. Meanwhile, in order to sleep and heal, you are better off with the *least* amount of stress hormones. If you are stressing yourself out at the end of a day, you're setting yourself up for lower-quality sleep.

Think of it this way: One of the times in our life that we tend to sleep the most is when we're growing up during infancy and childhood. After that, we get used to a lesser amount of sleep for a few years. Then puberty and the teenage years hit, and all we want to do is sleep again. We need sleep when we're teenagers because our bodies are evolving during that period our lives and need extra time to heal. There are pictures of me in my high school yearbook sleeping on a desk during class. I think I was drooling on a desk in one photo. Is this because I was a bad student? No—it's simply because teenagers aren't supposed to wake up at 6:30 a.m. to go to school. It may be necessary to make our lives fit a schedule so the world can be organized, but it would be fantastic if we could choose our own schedules for our whole lives based on what we need. When thinking about your sleep rules, keep this in mind: *Sleep equals healing.*

> **RULE:**
>
> Sleep = healing. Sleep six to nine hours a night.

Improve Quality of Sleep

Now that we've discussed *why* we need sleep, let's talk about optimum sleep positions to get the best sleep possible. If you're not sleeping in the right positions, you can put unnecessary stress on your body.

The only way *not* to sleep is on your stomach. If you're one of the unlucky small percentage of the population that sleep on their stomachs—well, even if you *occasionally* sleep on your stomach—*please, stop it!* For your sake, please stop. Next to jumping out of an airplane without a parachute, sleeping on your stomach is probably the single worst thing that you can do to your spine. Think about it: Sleeping on your stomach means you're spending hours at a time with your head turned to the side, twisting your spine and your muscles. What's worse, you probably turn to one side much more than the other, creating huge imbalances. The position of lying on your stomach with your head turned places stress on many of the nerves exiting your neck that travel to and communicate with the muscles going into your arms and hands. Those same nerves also branch off and travel to organs like your heart and lungs.

If people truly understood what they were doing when stomach-sleeping I'm sure they would stop, but it's not easy. Breaking the habit of stomach sleeping is like quitting smoking: You want to, but you're addicted to it. One of the best ways to stop is through understanding how it may be hurting you. As a chiropractor, I can tell you firsthand how much stress it's causing. If it's hard for you to stop sleeping on your stomach, the best thing to do is to try turning yourself into a side-sleeper first. The best way to sleep is on your back, but very few people can make the transition straight from stomach-sleeper to back-sleeper. Personally, I'm a side sleeper. The only times in my life when I've been a back sleeper were after breaking my back (twice), and after shoulder surgery. I experienced many nights of misery and frustration before I would finally pass out on my back from exhaustion. I do know how challenging it is to change your sleep habits. Start with sleeping on your side first.

I don't know many people who do sleep on their backs, but if you do, the proper pillow technique is to have one firm pillow under your head that supports the natural curve of your neck and doesn't allow your head to be pushed forward too far.

If you're still using your grandmother's soft, fluffy pillow, *get rid of it now*. It may have been okay to use thirty years ago, but pillows aren't built to last forever. When lying on your back, it's also a good idea to keep a pillow under your knees. The size depends on your comfort level; just a few inches of bend in the knees is sufficient.

Most of us sleep on our sides. To make lying on your side as comfortable as possible, I recommend the three pillow technique. The first pillow, for under your head, should be similar to the one I described for lying on your back: There should be enough support that your head doesn't sink too far into the pillow, and it should also not be so big that it pushes your head away too far.

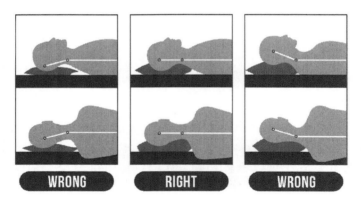

Second, you should have a pillow for in between your knees so they're not knocking together and so that there is something there to prevent you from rolling onto your belly.

Third, and most importantly, every side sleeper needs a hugger. If you're one of those people who is comfortable hugging your spouse or partner or dog all night, then kudos to you, but most of us can't sleep with all that extra body heat next to us. The perfect solution is a body pillow. The

purpose of this one is to keep your shoulders from cav
on each other while you're sleeping. This also helps you
if you like to sleep on your stomach because it puts a lit
pressure on your belly and makes you feel secure.

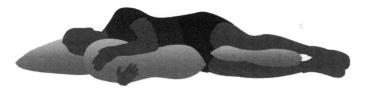

One last tidbit about sleep positioning: Switch sides of
the bed more often. If you share a bed with someone, you
typically wind up sleeping on the same side over and over
again. As a result, you also end up sleeping on the same side
of your body over and over again. If you're a side-sleeper
(like most of us), the tendency is to face the edge of the bed
and keep your back to the center of the bed. This is a more
secure position that innately enables us to not worry about
falling out of bed. Switch sides of the bed every two to three
months. It may feel weird at first, but believe me, you will
get used to it.

> **RULE:**
>
> Use proper pillow techniques and switch sides
> of the bed often. The pillow I recommend most
> these days? www.mypillow.com

Are You Having Trouble Sleeping?

Can't sleep? You may be having one of two problems.
- You can't fall asleep
- You can't stay asleep

The suggestions in this section will help you with both. Take what works for you and make rules for yourself around them!

If you can't fall asleep or stay asleep because you're physically uncomfortable, then you need to put down this book and make an appointment with your chiropractor, *right now*. Structural issues might be preventing you from being able to get physically comfortable in bed. You can also find out from your chiropractor how to exercise and stretch properly. It's also possible that a new bed is in your future—one uncomfortable spring can ruin your sleep.

Other places to look if you can't fall asleep or stay asleep are your grades in *Diet* and *Supplements*. Try cleaning up your diet by following the suggestions we talked about in that section. Add in the supplements that your health practitioner personally recommends for *you*. These are some of my general suggestions:

CALCIUM LACTATE

I recommend you get this from a company called Standard Process. Start with 250 mg before bed. Ever hear of drinking warm milk before bed? Milk upsets my stomach, which is why I recommend calcium lactate—it's not from milk. It's actually a vegetable source of calcium with a 5:1 ratio of calcium to magnesium. Drinking warm milk either works because it fills you up and makes you tired or the calcium and magnesium allow your brain to stop racing. Either way, I have seen a six-dollar bottle of calcium lactate get many a patient to sleep at night.

MELATONIN

Melatonin is a hormone secreted by our pineal gland. It helps regulate our sleep/wake cycles. I usually refrain from prescribing supplements that are an "end product." What is an end product? It's something that your body should be making on its own. From years of working with people, I usually see that if you get a person all of the required nutrients the body needs to make an end product, then it will. I don't believe there is a substitute for our body's own innate intelligence. It should know exactly how much melatonin to make, as long as it has all the raw ingredients and is put in the right environment. I don't particularly love prescribing nutrients that our bodies have the ability to create on their own, but this supplement (hormone) does work. What I've seen throughout the years, however, is that it only tends to work for relatively short periods of time. It's different for everyone, though.

GABA

GABA is a neurotransmitter (a chemical messenger for your nervous system). Its job is to be the "James Taylor" of neurotransmitters. It allows your brain to calm, chill out, and stop racing with thoughts. Your body produces GABA, so it is another one of those end products. There are many reasons why GABA may not be produced in the right quantities for some people. Since I don't like to prescribe end products, the best thing to do is take a supplement that stimulates your body's natural ability to produce more GABA. I usually recommend a blend of some vitamins, amino acids, and herbs that help the body produce GABA on its own. Keep in mind that when I recommend GABA support, I believe it should be done with the recommendation of a health practitioner. Currently, I use either Trancor from Metagenics or GabaFlow, Gabatone, or GabaCore from Apex Energetics. They all work differently, and I need different ones at different times.

By the way, be careful about buying any supplement called "GABA." GABA itself, as an end product, is practically useless. As mentioned previously in this book, GABA molecules are too large to be able to cross the blood/brain barrier. What that means is that if you take in GABA and feel more relaxed and have better sleep, it's either because of a placebo effect or because you have a "leaky brain." Leaky gut is described in a later chapter. Leaky brain is similar. There is supposed to be a barrier that keeps toxins or unwanted nutrients from crossing into the fluid-filled area that surrounds your brain and spinal cord. If that barrier is worn down, then these irritants can cross the barrier and affect your brain.

Again, I strongly recommend that you only try GABA-related supplements while under the care of a knowledgeable health provider. Don't mess with your brain chemistry on your own.

HERBS: CHAMOMILE, LAVENDER, AND LEMON BALM

Herbs are very effective at helping with sleep. You can get them in supplement form or simply drink them as a tea. Having a warm drink before bed is also very soothing and can relax you in its own right.

To repeat a recommendation I've already given you throughout this book so far, get to a great applied kinesiology doctor, functional medicine practitioner, naturopathic doctor, acupuncturist, or nutritionist to help determine which supplements are best for *you*.

To help you sleep better, look to improve your grade in *Exercise* as well by following the recommendations I gave you in that section. As you're probably already starting to see, *everything's connected.* You'll find that if you raise your grades in the areas of *Diet*, *Supplements*, and *Exercise*, you'll have an easier time falling asleep. If you haven't yet, read the chapter about exercise and make it a part of your life. If you want to get rid of your sleep problems, a long, physically demanding day or an exhausting workout might be just what you need for restful sleep.

In addition to improving your grades in all areas of your life and trying the recommendations above, I would highly recommend creating a ritual around sleep. Recall from Chapter 7 that a ritual is a set of habits put together in a sequence. Create a set of habits that you move through every night at the same time. As you move through your nighttime ritual each night, your body will naturally prepare itself for sleep. Make the time that you go to bed every night be part of your ritual—go to bed at the same time every night and wake up at the same time every morning. Here are some things I would recommend putting into your nighttime routine.

JOURNAL BEFORE BED

One reason people find it hard to fall asleep is because their minds are racing. Sometimes, it's hard to get your mind to slow down and relax after a busy day. You need to write down every mind-racing thought about the past day, the next day, and even far off into the future. Get it out of your head and onto paper. That way, you can rest easy knowing you can look at later and you won't forget anything. Now that you feel secure that you won't forget your crazy thoughts, you can fall asleep in peace (more on journaling in Chapter 16).

MEDITATE

I'll take you through meditation in detail a little later in this book (Chapter 16).

TURN OFF YOUR ELECTRONICS

Don't use electronics for at least half an hour before you go to bed. The flashing of lights—especially if you're watching TV with commercials flashing different attention-grabbing scenes—stimulates a dopamine reaction in your brain that is excitatory and can keep you awake. Put electronics like your computer and your phone away. Instead, get your mind into something simple like a book.

PROGRAM YOUR DREAMS

Tell yourself what you'd like to dream about. Start thinking about that for five or even fifteen minutes. Just spend some time thinking about that—you'd be surprised how much it can relax you.

If, after trying all of this, you're still having trouble sleeping, get to a sleep clinic or a mental health professional. I recommend this as a last resort, not because they don't know what they are doing—they are likely much more knowledgeable about sleep than I will ever be—but simply because that's not the point of this book. The point of using this book is to learn simple habits that hopefully replace the need for medications. If that doesn't work, then by all means, medicine may be a lifesaver.

> **RULE:**
>
> Sleep is a time to rest, repair, and heal. If you're having trouble sleeping, improve your grades in all areas of your life and create and follow a nighttime ritual. If you're still having trouble sleeping, get to a sleep clinic to improve your quality of sleep.

Chapter 13

Hydration

Why should we have a great grade in *Hydration*? Because at least 50 percent and up to 65 percent of our body is made of water. This one's pretty easy! Drink more water!

But sometimes it's not that easy! Some of you drink enough. Some people hold onto water better than others. The truth is that some of you are camels and some are thirsty dogs. One way I assess hydration in my office is by performing a test called a bioimpedance analysis. This test will calculate the total hydration of your body and will also calculate whether or not that water is getting into your cells or if it's floating around in your bloodstream.

We all need water in both compartments—intracellular, meaning inside your cells, and extracellular, meaning floating around our bloodstream—but the ratios change as we age. Think of it this way: Babies are *juicy*. We want to squeeze their cheeks and "take a bite out of them." Ninety-year-old people are simply *not juicy*. They may be cute, but they're not *juicy*. We all will wrinkle and shrivel as we age, so we want to preserve our large, juicy, young cells as long as we can. A bioimpedance analysis can give you a measurement of how young and juicy your cells are. I use this measurement to monitor my recommendations for nutrition and lifestyle advice in my office. If the plan you are on is making your cells bigger and juicier, then it's most likely the right plan. If it isn't, then we adjust it.

In general, you can get your cells more hydrated (juicy) by optimizing your percentage of muscle, by improving the quality of foods and/or supplements you are ingesting, or by making sure that you are absorbing those nutrients by improving your digestive health. You can also decrease the toxins in your body to get more water into your cells (see section on detoxing in Chapter 20).

In terms of how much water to drink, let's say you aren't a patient at my office and your doctor doesn't do bioimpedance analysis or coach you in cellular hydration. Simply try this rule: Drink half your weight in fluid ounces of water each day.

How do you make sure you do that? I'm really busy most workdays, so I have to plan how I drink water. I want to get about seventy-five ounces a day, but I don't have time to run to the bathroom and pee all throughout the day, so here's what I do: I drink a large glass of water every morning with my supplements, I have a few more ounces before I leave my car and walk into the office, I drink very little most of the day (except when I work out), and then I drink about thirty-five to forty ounces on my hour-long drive home. Sure, I listen to my body as well. If I'm thirsty, I drink water, but I make sure that I have my rules for when the optimal time is for me to drink, so I never go too far off track. When you're busy, you sometimes just "forget" to drink. My rules help me to do better!

Hydration doesn't simply mean water! Now that you've got the water part down, let's take a moment to discuss electrolytes. Electrolytes are the nutrients/chemicals that are vital for many functions, including the ability for your muscles to contract and relax properly (remember, your heart is a muscle). The major electrolytes include calcium, magnesium, potassium, and even sodium (salt). There are others that are all easy to assess from a medical standpoint. A simple blood test will do. We're not talking about severe deficiency of electrolytes here, though; we're talking about simple ways to measure whether you're at optimal levels.

My favorite self-analysis tool is to assess muscle cramping. If your toes, feet, or calves cramp occasionally in the middle of the night or with heavy activity, you may need to increase the amount of electrolytes you ingest. You should be able to get the electrolytes you need from a great diet, but if you don't have an A yet, you may need a supplement. Also, if you're an athlete, pushing your body hard or exercising in hot weather or in a hot yoga class, your demand for electrolytes may be greater than the average Joe!

Which minerals do you need? How much do you need? I would say it's different for everyone, but as soon as you get the right mix, your foot and toe cramps should disappear! My best recommendation, of course, is to find a health practitioner who can guide you through the process of figuring out what supplement is best for you but, most likely, the recommendation *won't* be for more Gatorade or some sweet sports drink! At least not from me. *There are exceptions*, but I don't believe that most people need high amounts of sugars, artificial sweeteners, or artificial colors and flavors to fulfill their hydration requirements.

Most of the foods we eat contain electrolytes, so why would we need more? I'll refer you to my earlier survive/thrive point. Unless I am working with a patient who is very ill, lab tests don't usually reveal an electrolyte deficiency. I do often see patients who cramp or have their muscles twitch during exercise. These symptoms may only be occasional, but it could be a sign that they are not eating enough good, high-quality food. It could also be that they are not absorbing nutrients properly. One common reason for malabsorption can be medications. Proton pump inhibitors for acid reflux, for example, can impact our ability to absorb electrolytes.

The simplest recommendation I can make to improve your electrolyte status is to introduce some coconut water into your life. Coconut water is a great natural source of electrolytes, and nowadays, it can be found all over the place. Your body should provide clear feedback on how much is right for you. Too much, and you may feel your stomach upset or notice changes in your bowel movements. The right amount will help to quench your thirst, and you should see those cramps disappear!

RULE:

Drink half your body weight in fluid ounces of water a day. If you're still thirsty because of a hot day or a hard workout, drink additional water or add coconut water. To avoid constant bathroom breaks, set up the optimal times throughout your day to drink water.

Chapter 14

Alignment and Posture

Part 1: What's So Important about Posture?

Let's begin with a *why*. Why should we even pay attention to alignment and posture in the first place? There are many reasons why, but my favorite explanation is that your posture and how you carry yourself in this world is a reflection of who you are as a person and how you project yourself to others.

Try this exercise: Close your eyes (not just yet, first read the instructions) and imagine a person in your mind. This person represents the epitome of health and wellness. This person is incredibly successful and confident in their own skin. This person is friendly, kind, compassionate, and leads others to be better than they are. How does this person carry themselves? Do they slouch, or do they stand tall? Do their shoulders round forward, or do they naturally seem to be in line with the rest of their body?

What sort of image did you get? Maybe you pictured a person you know, or maybe you pictured a fictitious superhero. Let's do the exercise again. This time, close your eyes and picture a person who stands before you that is unhealthy. They just don't feel great. This person is stressed out and doesn't feel confident around others. This person is kind and compassionate as well but keeps to themselves

ιe time. Do you picture the same person in your
d they take on a different posture?

ve choose to carry ourselves is also what we project
ιeople around us. It's what makes us "attractive."
ιat word in quotes because I am not describing beau-
ty-contest attractive, I am describing the most powerful
type of attractive—the kind of people who we are drawn
to because they possess a certain energy that we like to be
around. Sure, great looks help a lot. If you are lucky enough
to be born with beauty, you happen to have an upper hand
in this world. But personally, I've met some very "unat-
tractive" good-looking people in my day.

So, how do we become more attractive? Well, posture is
a great place to start. What if you don't feel attractive right
now? Then fake it! "Fake it 'til you make it" is the expression, isn't it? Carry yourself tall and with confidence—not
rigid and upright and cocky, but tall and confident. Even
when you don't feel it, you will still project that energy to
others. I believe you'll also project it out to the universe.

There's a fantastic TED talk about posture that I believe
everyone should watch at least once. Search for "Amy Cud-
dy: Your body language shapes who you are." This twen-
ty-one-minute talk sums up what I want to convey.

Let me give you another reason why alignment and posture are so important. Let's do another visualization exercise. I want you to think of two eighty-seven-year-old people. One needs a walker to get around and complains about
all of the aches and pains of aging. The other is still playing
tennis three times a week, goes on long hikes, and enjoys
playing with their great-grandkids. We've all seen or know
someone representative of both types.

What is the difference between these two people? Usually, it's their lifestyle. The lifestyle of the active, life-loving
eighty-seven-year-old probably includes diet and exercise

and the right mindset about life. I believe those are vital aspects of health, and they're all taught in this book. But the one aspect that most people disregard is their *alignment*, simply because people don't understand the importance. And even if people do the important, many don't think there's anything they can do about it.

Below are a few examples of good versus poor alignment.

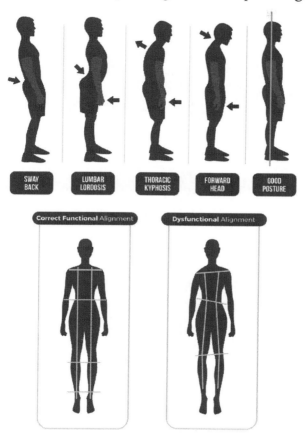

The basics are as follows. From the side view, your ear, shoulder, hip, knee, and ankle should all fall along the same line. From the front or back view, your ears, shoulders, and hips should all be level, and your feet should have a mild flare, pointing in the same direction.

If you are living with postural imbalances like to ones described and depicted above, then the forces of gravity are simply weighing more heavily on you. A body out of alignment experiences more stress than a body in alignment. Plain and simple. So, if the goal is to be healthy, and one aspect of health is making sure we address the physical stress that is wearing us down, then we need to get our posture and alignment as correct as they can be. A body with poor alignment experiences more stress and wears down faster than a body with great alignment.

Keep in mind that these are examples of *optimal* alignment and posture. You don't have to have a perfect posture to be healthy, but it helps to be as close to optimal as your body will allow.

I have a patient named Lisa. Lisa has scoliosis. She first came to me at the age of twenty-eight. By that age, it is very difficult to completely correct scoliosis of the spine. What did I do with Lisa, then? We got her better! You see, Lisa's version of an A+ posture was different than most. I gave her a grade of an A+ after her posture improved as far as we thought it could. She still had a high right shoulder, and her mid-back arched forward, but that was the best she could have achieved, given what scoliosis had done to her spine over the course of twenty-eight years of her life. Remember, the goal is better, not perfect. Lisa eats well, exercises regularly, meditates, loves her job and her family, and, in general, has many other great health grades. As a result, I believe the effects of her scoliosis will be minimal.

Improve Your Posture

So, how do you raise your grade in the area of alignment and posture? You *must* exercise. The more toned and fit you are muscle-wise, the better your posture will be.

Recall from the chapter on *Exercise* that the key is to ensure that you're working out properly. I want you to make sure that you are exercising *all* your muscles—not *just* running or *only* doing push-ups and sit-ups or *only* being active by playing tennis.

You should be striving to make sure that you're stimulating *every single part of your body equally.* The best way to do that is to find a great personal trainer, take a bunch of classes, or exercise with a great set of videos. Again, just like I mentioned in the *Exercise* section, personal, one-on-one training is ideal. Group classes are the second-best, and videos or books are a great resource after that.

The alignment of your posture will change as you develop your muscles properly. Build proper muscle tone, as I mentioned in the section on *Body Composition.* I would also recommend stretching often in order to enable your muscles to adequately support your structural balance. Stretching keeps muscles *flexible* and strong. The absolute best tool for learning how to stretch is to start taking yoga classes. I thought I knew how to stretch before I began my weekly yoga class. Now I get to enjoy the benefits of great stretching and also spend an hour a week working on the symmetry and tone of my body in a completely different way than I have in the past.

Do you want to learn how to stretch but don't want to do yoga? By now, you probably know what I'm going to suggest! Google the word "stretch" and click on a video that suits your needs.

Here's another quick practice you can use at home or work to help you take care of one of the most important parts of your physical body contributing to your alignment: your feet.

Keep a Tennis Ball under Your Desk

Here's a simple rule to help your feet. Keep a tennis ball under your desk at work. Don't have a desk? Keep one anywhere you sit down regularly, where it won't interfere with the rest of your life—maybe on the floor in the kitchen isn't such a good idea, for example! Why keep a tennis ball close at hand? Because our feet take a beating!

How many steps have you taken? I don't just mean today. How many steps have you taken *ever*? Stress is cumulative. Over the course of our lives, our feet are very good to us, but if we don't care for them, they eventually start to hurt. Pamper those feet of yours by rolling your foot over a tennis ball once a day for one minute per foot. Roll back and forth, side to side, and in little circles to make a pattern. It's like giving yourself a foot massage every day. It's better to use a ball rather than a wooden, dowel type of device, in my opinion—you want it to be something that will roll away from you if you don't pay a bit of attention to it. This creates a higher mind-body connection because you have to control the ball with your mind—not merely your foot.

> **RULE:**
>
> Kick off your shoes once a day and roll your feet over a tennis ball.

In addition to stretching and taking care of your feet to improve your posture, it's important to be aware of how you're carrying yourself during all activities throughout your day. The way you carry yourself means something, and it has an impact on your alignment. How can you improve how you carry yourself? Google "How do I improve my posture" and select the video section. Here, you will find

193,000 results, at my last check—chiropractors, physical therapists, and yoga instructors—all teaching great ways to improve posture. Of course, I'm biased toward the chiropractic videos, mostly because we've been doing it the longest. But overall, you'll find a wealth of information on the internet.

The most important thing is to start. Get going on this, *now*. If you see your posture improving, great. If not, move on to the next video and take the next piece of advice. Overall, over the course of your lifetime, you should be working on achieving an A in *Posture and Alignment* because it's going to improve your life in tremendous ways, now and especially in your future.

I want this book to be a tool to remind you of what you should be doing, and I can't fit all the information on improving posture in these pages! There's simply too much.

Chapter 15

Alignment and Posture

Part 2: The Basics of Chiropractic Care

There is no better-suited health practitioner to help you achieve the alignment and posture you are looking for than a good chiropractor.

I want you to know that I wrote and rewrote this section at least a dozen times. The version that you are about to read was written just a few days before I sent my book out for its final edit. Why did I have such a hard time? Because I could not possibly convey the importance of chiropractic care in just one section of one book. What I will do here is teach you that a good chiropractor is the best doctor to help you if you want good alignment and posture. I'll also explain the kind of chiropractic care practiced in my office.

Chiropractic in a Nutshell

The chiropractic adjustment, done properly, is the single most efficient tool for removing the damaging effects of stress on the body.

The words "done properly" in the sentence above refers to the fact that every person has different needs. The same adjustment to the spine can have an incredibly powerful, positive effect on one person, yet have no effect at all on someone else. This is the best explanation for why there are millions of people who love their chiropractors. At the same time, there is a relatively small amount of double-blind, placebo-controlled research that substantiates what we do. I hope I haven't just created some enemies out of fellow chiropractors out there, but this book is based on twenty-five years of experience in the chiropractic profession. We are much more effective than our research can show.

Chiropractic is a science, but it is also a philosophy and an art. There have been many scientific studies touting the benefits of chiropractic care, but the studies done so far haven't really been able to encompass the full benefits of having a chiropractor on your team of health professionals. Why? Maybe it's because what I do—and what many chiropractors do—simply cannot be studied very easily. That's because chiropractic is also a philosophy and an art; what happens in an office, with a real patient in front of you, is often different than an encounter during a study.

The Philosophy

The premise of chiropractic philosophy states that there is a universal intelligence in all matter. In living organisms, it is called *innate intelligence.* This innate intelligence controls and coordinates all of the subconscious functions of our bodies, allowing us to heal and remain healthy. The *expression* of this intelligence, however, can be interfered with. The goal of the chiropractor is to remove interference so the body can heal.

Chiropractic has not survived over 120 years because we're good at relieving lower back pain. People who visit chiropractors regularly, at least in some way, understand that their chiropractor helps to keep them healthy overall. How? By simply removing stress on their bodies so they don't have to be burdened by the effects.

Less stress on the body means improved health. I truly believe that when each person can simply understand that one point, we are healthier! We are better when we are well-aligned and carrying less physical stress. Then we can appreciate chiropractic care.

The Art

To provide a glimpse of this art, I thought I would walk you through a typical patient visit as seen through the eyes of the artist. There are over one hundred different techniques in the chiropractic profession. I am a practitioner of applied kinesiology, so what you are about to read will be the encounter as it happens through my eyes. There are many other unique ways to get to the same end result: a healthy patient.

The main quality you should look for when choosing a practitioner is their innate desire to help you. Personally, I feel that applied kinesiology offers the practitioner the most insight into helping a patient get better, but there are no wrong ways of practicing chiropractic. Also, each practitioner will bring their own experiences and wisdom to each and every technique, therefore making it their own.

A Patient Visit through Dr. Piken's Eyes

I first see you in the reception area and ask you to come back to the adjusting room. Your visit really started though as soon as you walked in the door—heck, as soon as you scheduled your visit, the care really begins. Before you even enter the office, the chiropractic artist has made sure that their team of "front-of-the-house" caregivers is thinking about you and how they can better serve you. This means that the first part of your adjustment is the way you are welcomed into the practice.

Next, from the first second I see you, I am reading you. I want to see how you get up from the chair, how you walk back to the adjustment room, what you choose to say or not say. Whether you feel like sitting or if you allow me to guide you directly into a posture check. As I look at your posture, I'm not merely looking for the high shoulder or the tilted pelvis or pronated foot or head tilt. I'm letting your body "speak." If I give it just enough time—maybe even while we're talking about how you feel or some insignificant topic like the weather—I'm really getting information. You will tell me with your body, not your words, where the most important area of stress is and where I should continue to evaluate. It may be your foot, your shoulder, your neck... . It may or may not be the directly symptomatic area you are feeling at that moment, but it's the most important area to assess because it's what your body communicated to me in the first place.

From there, we usually begin the communication known as manual muscle testing. Manual muscle testing is a technique that can be used to isolate and determine how each muscle in the body is functioning. The purpose of muscle testing is not purely mechanistic; it's not about whether the muscle is testing at a four out of five, a five out of five, or—and I really hope not—a three out of five. It's a conversation that I have with your body. I'm asking, "Is there 100 percent function here? How about here? Well, how about over here?" I'm listening as to whether your muscles are functioning to the best of their ability. You just have to let me ask and be open to your body's answer.

This is confusing to some people at first, but most patients understand it over the course of a few visits, as trust is built between us. During a muscle test, a perfect score of five out of five either means that the muscle is 100 percent connected (the most common reason), or it could mean that you're not ready to let go of your tension and really show me where the problem is. The desire to win or the fear of being weak can interfere with the test because, ultimately, I can only listen to what your body allows me to pick up.

Once a weak or disconnected muscle is discovered, the next part of our conversation—or our "dance," as I like to think of the art of applied kinesiology—is to determine the cause of that weakness. I will touch or I will have you touch areas of your body that correlate with nerve, neurolymphatic, neurovascular, acupunctural, emotional, or nutritional reflex points and look to see what makes you "stronger." Based on the positions I place you in or the reflex points I have you touch, muscles will seem to magically become weaker or stronger. This test is giving me feedback about what's working for you and what isn't. My best recommendation is to simply let go and allow the conversation to happen.

I know that many people will have a hard time understanding this concept by simply reading about it. I would recommend seeking a certified practitioner to learn more. As long as your applied kinesiology practitioner has the *intent* of helping you, and you trust in their intent, please let down your guard and let the conversation flow.

At this point, we've found the part of the body that needs help, and we've also found the reflexes that need to be corrected to allow you to heal. What does that mean? What we are looking for are *subluxations*.

The Subluxation: The Principle of Chiropractic

Technically, the term "vertebral subluxation" means a misalignment of the spine that is interfering with the nervous system by inducing stress. To me, a subluxation does not have to be spinal. A subluxation is any physical, chemical, emotional stress that is keeping you from expressing your best self. The adjustment—or correction—is the clearing of the subluxation or the removal of whatever is preventing you from being your best self. The last part of your visit is all about correcting what we have found.

The premise of all chiropractic is this: We have an incredible, *innate* ability to heal. That ability *never* ceases. It is always available to us; we are constantly growing new cells to repair our bodies. We have been doing it since conception, and the same ability to heal is with us throughout our entire lives. The subluxation, however, interferes with that expression of innate wisdom and the ability to heal.

Subluxations can be physical, as in a misaligned spine, a knot in a muscle, or tension and scar tissue in your fascia. Subluxations can be chemical: something unwanted or unneeded that you are eating/ingesting, smelling/inhaling, or rubbing on your body, producing inflammation or causing your body to work harder. Or subluxations can be emotional: a thought that you can't get rid of because of a conversation five minutes ago at work, or the ways you've been conditioned to think, thanks to the people who raised you. "Subluxation" is merely a word referring to something that is stressing your body and interfering with your ability to express 100 percent health.

After we find your subluxation or subluxations, the next step is easy. We correct them. At our office, the correction might be a chiropractic adjustment to the spine, specific types of soft tissue work, therapeutic laser, exercises, teaching you how to meditate, teaching you what to eat, advising what supplements to take ... and more.

Many people think chiropractors are exclusively back pain and neck pain doctors, but there is a difference between chiropractic as an *art* and chiropractic as pain management. If all you desire is increased range of motion and some temporary relief from pain, then there are plenty of great chiros out there to help you naturally eliminate aches and pains. But if what you are looking for is an expert in the body who can guide you to understand how to truly be healthy, then find an applied kinesiology practitioner or a principled chiropractor—or both—who will teach you what it truly means to be healthy.

I have an amazing job. It's my calling, and it is a constantly rewarding way to spend my day. I get to look at the incredible puzzle of the human being in front of me and try to *figure them out*. That's it.... I am not just trying to increase their range of motion or make them feel better, as much as I do love when those things happen. My ultimate goal is to help my patients evolve and transform into the best possible versions of themselves. I do this by removing interference from their bodies by adjusting their spines, working on their muscles, showing them how to move better, and encouraging them to put nourishing foods into their bodies nourishing thoughts into their minds. If you allow your chiropractor and or practitioner of applied kinesiology to work with you, you will have found the greatest doctor on the planet. After all, the word *doctor* means "to teach." If you are lucky enough to find a chiropractor/practitioner of applied kinesiology who will learn what your body is trying to say—and who will teach you what he or she finds—then you'll live a life with less stress and less interference. Your innate potential can be expressed to its fullest.

One last point about chiropractic: If you haven't found the right chiropractor to work with you, keep looking. Remember, there are many ways to practice chiropractic, just like there are many specialties in medicine. Don't base your opinion on what chiropractors can do for you during one visit to one office—or, even worse, based on what someone else said. Find out for yourself.

RULE:

Find an applied kinesiologist or a chiropractor who practices the *art* of chiropractic.

Chapter 16

Stress Management

Wе all have emotional stress in our lives. In fact, we either have stress, or we're dead. The only people who don't have any stress whatsoever are non-living.

That being said, there are different levels of emotional stress, and when it goes out of control in any way, shape, or form, either because you're taking on too much or you're not handling it well, things go awry in the body and something happens. Stress is like calories. If you eat more calories than you burn, you gain weight, and after weeks, months, or years of your calorie equation being out of balance (more calories in than out), you can see the damaging effects on your body.

Every day, we are exposed to combinations of physical, chemical, and emotional stress—that's inevitable. But if we do little to alleviate the stress we experience, we throw off the balance in our stress equation. The effects of stress aren't as quickly apparent as calories, but they do impact our health in a tremendously negative way.

Stress can trigger the body's response to perceived threats or dangers: the fight-or-flight response. During this reaction, certain hormones like adrenaline and cortisol are released, speeding the heart rate, slowing digestion, shunting blood flow to major muscle groups, and changing various other autonomic nervous functions. In the moment, this gives the body a burst of energy to be able to deal with the threat at hand. When the perceived threat is gone, systems are designed to return to normal function via the relaxation response, but in our times of chronic stress, this often doesn't happen enough. Therefore, the stress we endure causes damage to the body.

So how do you manage the inevitable stress that will come your way on a day-to-day basis? How can you raise your grade in this area?

Here is the list of habits, rules, and rituals that you need to make part of your daily life to minimize the effects of emotional stress. Keep in mind, as always, that you don't need to implement *all* these strategies at once. The best way to improve your grades without creating *more* stress is to pick the one that innately gets you excited and you feel can turn into a habit or ritual the easiest. Once that *one thing* is mastered and a regular part of your life—I don't care whether it takes a few days, a few weeks, or a few months to implement—if you feel your grade is still not an A, then you're ready to add another tool. Try some of these strategies to help you improve your grade in *Stress Management*.

YOUR MORNING RITUAL

In the beginning of this book, we spoke about your morning ritual, or setting the tone for the day, as having the greatest impact on how you handle your stress throughout the day. Your morning ritual will set you up in the best possible way to manage the stress of the day ahead. Here's a quick refresher of what that can look like:

- Wake up, and as soon as you can, begin the day with prayer and/or gratefulness. Here's where I'll advise you to go back to Chapter 6 and reread the sections on setting the tone of the day with prayer and gratefulness.

- Exercise—Refer back to the section on exercise. Exercise is one of the single *best forms of stress relief* in the world.

- Meditation is also one of the *best* forms of stress relief. You have to find at least five minutes a day—ideally, twenty minutes, twice per day—to meditate. See the section on *Meditation* for more on this.

- You can't forget *sex!* I could not possibly leave out one of the *best* forms of stress relief here (I hope no instruction is needed for this recommendation).

- Journaling—Even though this can be used as a great part of your morning ritual, I also often recommend to my patients that journaling can be done before bed. It is great for clearing your mind and relieving stress.

How to Journal

There are many ways to implement any of the suggestions in this book. As far as journaling goes, here is my favorite recommendation. Before bed, write down your list of *must-dos* for tomorrow and set aside five minutes of free-writing. One of the many things that affect our ability to handle stress is our ability to get quality sleep. There is an entire section on sleep in the book, but journaling is a crossover recommendation that helps your *Stress Management*, *Sleep*, and *Connectedness* grades. I decided it would be best placed here.

One of the reasons why we have trouble sleeping is because our minds race around with too many thoughts about the future. So one simple technique that will make things *better* is to write down a list of everything that you must do the next day to simply get it out of your head.... If you take this one minute to jot down a list for the next day, your mind will be at bit more at ease. You won't have to have that loop spinning around in your head about making sure to "pack the kids' lunches" ... or make sure you remember your gym bag ... or that one detail in the report that you just thought about just as you got into bed... . Just write it down and get it out. There's something cathartic about putting pen to paper—something permanent and tangible. So write it down and stare at it. This isn't a big, long goal planning session—just get out the essentials. It should only take a minute.

Next, take another five minutes to free-write! Thank you, Mr. Shapiro! He was an English teacher I had in twelfth grade who introduced me to the process of free-writing. I love it. Very simply put, free-writing is this: Get a pen and some paper, preferably a nice journal book, and once you place the tip of the pen to the paper and begin writing, *do not stop!* Seriously. Keep writing no matter what! I don't care if you're scribbling, not writing, blah, blah, blah... . Keep writing whatever thought pops into your head. After a few seconds, thoughts and words will form and *don't stop!* If you can't write fast enough to keep up with the thoughts in your head, no worries. It doesn't need to be legible. You never really have to read it again. The point is that you're getting your thoughts out so they aren't *stuck* in your head to review over and over again.

Here are a few tips for your journaling/free-writing. First, pen and paper—not electronic, if that's possible. Why wouldn't it be possible? Well, rule two: it needs to be confidential. You need to be able to feel safe with what you have written. You need to feel that there is no way that anyone else will ever read what you have written unless you want them to. If you can accomplish that with pen and paper and a drawer to slip it into when you're done because you completely trust the ones you live with, great. If you don't feel that secure, then you can easily secure an electronic version. Simply set up a couple new private e-mails and e-mail yourself every night before bed. Problem solved. I'm sure there are other solutions you could come up with as well. If thoughts are kept in your head that race around, preventing you from achieving quality sleep or handling stress, then you need to get those thoughts out!

Why only five minutes of free-writing? Well, if you want to write a book, go ahead! But five minutes every day is a great habit that you can implement right now.... . That's all you need! Below are some other suggestions for stress relief that you can implement throughout your day!

Take Breaks at Work

Taking breaks is a great way to relieve stress during your work day. Most people sit way too much! Sitting is great, but we've gotten to a point where we sit too much. Because of this, we have to follow this rule: *Get up and move!*

Our bodies are designed to move (recall the chapter on *Exercise*), but sitting at work is a necessary evil that most of us can't avoid. We sit at a desk or stand in one place for many hours a day in order to make a living. But the longer we sit, the longer we let stress accumulate in our bodies. So here are some suggestions for you to keep you moving during your day:

TAKE MICRO-BREAKS

Whether it's standing or walking every fifteen minutes, take micro-breaks. A perfect example is right now, as I was writing this. I was thinking of taking a micro-break, so I just did it! Really! I did! It only took seven seconds! I stood up, stretched backward, twisted back and forth, and arched my back! That's all a micro-break has to be.

I know it's difficult when you break your train of thought on a project, but believe me—you can hold that thought for an extra ten to twelve seconds if you really want to! A micro-break should be taken about every fifteen minutes or so—and take more, if you want! The more you move, the better. Don't use your micro-breaks as an excuse to do poor quality or slow-paced work; use them as a quick refuel so you'll actually be *more* productive. If you feel better because you're moving, you will make better decisions and get more done!

TAKE SHORT BREAKS EVERY HOUR ("ONE-HOUR BREAKS")

Every hour or so, you should also take an extended short break. Get a drink of water! Have a few cut-up veggies ... anything to get you moving. Keep it under five minutes. Get up and walk or stretch. Change your environment a bit. Again, use this little mental/spiritual/physical moment to reset and refresh.

EAT LUNCH AWAY FROM YOUR DESK!

Get up and get out! Leave your place of business for lunch and have a little enjoyment during your day. Sometimes, I only get fifteen minutes, but if that's all I get, then I would rather go out and get my own food and eat somewhere else in that fifteen minutes than sit at the place I sit all day long and not truly have a break. My lunch rule for timing is to take as long as you can while still getting your work done and *get out of your office!*

> **RULE:**
>
> Take breaks throughout your work day. Keep your body moving. Eat lunch away from your desk!

Overall, the best way to alleviate stress and its effects is to live a healthy lifestyle. You need proper rest, regular exercise, and excellent nutrition. As you bring up your marks in the other areas of your report card, you'll find that this mark will inevitably go up as well. Remember, stress is cumulative, just like calories—if it builds up for weeks, months, or even years, the effects add up and can compound. The healthier you are, the better you will be able to manage the inevitable stress that is part of life.

In addition to a healthy lifestyle, I now want to give you a few more habits you can implement to reduce stress in your life.

Other Ways to Reduce and Manage Stress

There are passive ways to help with stress. What "passive" means is that you're letting someone else help with your stress when you need a little extra help! Remember that there are three different kinds of stress: physical, emotional, and chemical. You could seek out chiropractic, massage, acupuncture, or even a good therapist, psychologist, or social worker to help with emotional stress.

And how about this?! *Have more freakin' fun!* Remember: Life is *too short.* Make sure you plan some time off from work. Plan more time with your family and friends. Enjoy yourself! No one ever claimed on their deathbed that they wished they had worked more hours—people usually look back and regret not enjoying life as much as they could have! Take a vacation every quarter—maybe it's a staycation or maybe it's only an extra-long weekend—but do something *different.* Just simply breaking your routine and stimulating the dopamine centers of your brain with a little fun and excitement goes a long way when you do it often enough. Try not to wait until your burnt out before you take the time to have fun.

Here are some other things you can do to reduce the amount of stress in your life:

- Read a book
- Take more time to enjoy the hobby
- Start enjoying a *new* hobby!
- Play with your kids! Read to your kids! Enjoy hobbies with your kids!
- Get a pet—hopefully a rescue—and take great care of them! Play with them. I have two rescued dogs who are two of the greatest joys in my life!

And finally, try this for stress relief:
Service! Service! Service!

There are few things in life that make you feel as good as helping others! I'm not simply talking about giving money (although that's great thing, too); I'm talking about spending some time—any amount of time—helping another human being or animal. This has been thoroughly researched as one of the greatest stress relievers! Find a soup kitchen, get involved with a local charity, or help out at your place of worship. The more you give, the better you're going to feel!

RULE:

Implement one new stress-reducing strategy each year and prioritize it.

WHY ZEBRAS DON'T GET ULCERS

Why Zebras Don't Get Ulcers, **by Robert Sapolsky, describes how the stress process works and how it relates to the human condition.**

Sapolsky spent months at a time, for years, living in the Serengeti and studying wildlife, specifically baboons. The baboons he studied lived in a protected wildlife preserve that had an abundance of food and water. They had no predators and no worries about food or shelter (they lived in the trees). It would seem that the baboons were completely stress-free. Wrong! Sapolsky found that the baboons, while they could have been living the greatest of stress-free lives, instead actually *created* stress amongst themselves. They would bicker and fight with each other and compete for "top baboon." They had no natural *external* sources of stress, so they *created* stress amongst themselves.

When I read Sapolsky's book, I kept thinking that it sounded like this preserve of baboons was a mix between corporate America and high school: cliques, power struggles, fights, family issues, conflicts with friends, and *ulcers*. In fact, the baboons suffered from a mix of things like ulcers, diabetes, arthritis and even cancer—diseases that humans experience and that are not readily seen in wildlife.

Contrast this story with that of zebras: Zebras *don't* get ulcers. They're lower on the food chain. Because they're prey and they know it—at least on some level—they stick together. Zebras don't get ulcers because the stress that they experience is the stress of life and death. They don't create the stress of *who's going to be the top baboon/football player/CEO?*

Overall, what Sapolsky found is that even though all of the above can be classified as *stress*, the type or kind of stress that we're exposed to *does* matter. We're affected by life and death stress differently than by stress that we create among our own species. It often takes a common threat of "the un-known" to bring us together. For example, think of the blackout of the summer of 2002 in the northeast part of the US. Because we weren't sure what was happening and we knew we were all affected, there was a sense of bonding and brotherhood/sister-hood. A lot of the self-imposed stress disappeared in those moments.

At the heart of it, we will create our own self-im-posed stress if we don't have to worry about the stress of survival. Understanding this reality can help us choose to dissolve the stress that we're cre-ating unnecessarily.

How are you creating self-imposed stress in your own life? I invite you to release it now!

Chapter 17

Connectedness

Given how fast-paced life is and how overstimulated we all are by social media and everything around us, it is becoming more and more important to have practices that keep us connected to *ourselves*. What does it mean to be connected to yourself? It means you always have a way to recharge and rejuvenate yourself, no matter how crazy life may get. Becoming *connected* is about finding your source of inner power by being *with yourself* and *by yourself.* This section is about going *within* to be able to connect better with yourself and the people around you.

Connectedness could mean connecting with your purpose or passion in life. It could mean truly connecting with those you love and the people around you. It could mean connecting with nature. It could mean connecting with religious principles that are meaningful to you. Whatever it means to you, connecting with *yourself* enables you to recharge your batteries and ground yourself with what's truly important to you, no matter what is happening in the busyness of day-to-day life.

Having a great grade in this area of your report card is very important because without a connection to yourself and those around you, you run the risk of ending up running around *doing* a bunch of things during your day without being present as to *why* you're doing them. We all need to stay grounded and connected to what really matters. You can eat well, exercise, drink enough water, keep your body structurally aligned, and manage your stress effectively—but if you're not grounded in who you *really* are and *what's import-ant to you* on a regular basis, you can burn out.

Try the simple techniques in this chapter to raise your grade in this area and stay grounded and connected to your infinite source of inner power and energy. Your connection to yourself will also reveal the starting points for truly connecting with others in your life—something that is immensely important to us as human beings.

Disconnect to Connect

I love the comedian Louis C.K. I find that he has a great ability to insert philosophy into comedy. I saw a great clip of him talking to Conan O'Brian. I've seen many great clips of him on Conan—look them up on YouTube. This particular one was about how we all are so obsessed with our cell phones and being constantly connected to everyone and everything around us.

I simply cannot do this issue justice on paper. We've probably all had thoughts like this before: *How much technology is too much? Are my kids texting too much? Am I texting too much? I can't help but look at my phone every time it beeps, yet I really want a break!*

While I do believe all this technology has its place, I will argue that it has actually *decreased* our ability to connect. Sure, because of technology, we can keep in touch with people we might not have in the past. It's easy now to send a quick "hello" and check out a pic or two on Facebook. But the trouble is that when we do reach out to people, the connection is like a quick sound bite rather than a connection that contributes to the fabric of true relationships. It's easy now to have a "sound bite relationship" with a lot of people. But, as humans, we all need—yes *need*—real, deep connections to other humans.

There's plenty of research that proves we are healthier and happier when we have people we consider close friends and family as a part of our lives. We produce more endorphins (our body's own natural, good-feeling chemicals) when we interact with those we care about. In fact, the more face-to-face time we spend with them—at least phone time, and maybe even some Facetime or Skype time—the better. Texting and e-mail just don't do it. Sure, every once in a while, an e-mail or a Facebook message can elicit an emotion, but we need to take more time to *fully connect*.

First, we all need to get more connected *in the relationships we have with ourselves.* Think of it—unless you happen to be a conjoined twin, you spend more time with yourself than any other person. You can't get away from yourself. Yet technology today has given us so many distractions and our lives are filled with so much stuff, information, planned activities, and options that we can easily disconnect from *ourselves.* We need to find a way to stop being distracted by everyone and everything around us and reconnect with ourselves.

One of the greatest ways of slowing down life and connecting with yourself is by spending twenty-four hours with *just yourself.* Realistically, we probably need a few days or a week by ourselves, but how about first trying twenty-four hours?

When was the last time you went twenty-four hours without communicating one word or one thought to another person or listening to any words or communications from another person? For most of us, it just doesn't happen. If you meditate like I do, then you're on your own for at least a few minutes a day, but try spending twenty-four hours alone. Just one day of your life in a state of *zero communication* can do wonders for you. You will get a lot out of it.

The best thing to do is to prepare for some alone time by letting all of your closest family and friends know that "Starting on Friday the ...., I will not be able to send or receive messages, contact you, or answer your calls ... nothing until the next night, Saturday the ...." Then get yourself prepped for your twenty-four hours. Turn off your cell phone, unplug your landline, and turn off your TV and computer. Put away all magazines and newspapers and do not listen to music. Write out a nice, clear note saying, *Sorry I cannot speak to you. I have extreme laryngitis, and I have been told by my doctor that I cannot even attempt to communicate with anyone until ___.* Carry it around with you, just in case someone comes to your door or bumps into you as you're walking wherever you're going that day. Just flash the paper for ten seconds and move on in silence.

During that time on your own, watch no movies. Preferably, you should also read no books, but I don't have a problem with reading a book on meditation, spirituality (whatever your expression of spirituality is), or religion. Just try not to read anything that may not be uplifting. Sometimes, religious books can be interpreted as someone else's rules set out for you to follow. These twenty-four hours are all about you, so choose what you read carefully. Journaling your thoughts would be a better option.

The day should be completely introspective, and you should allow your mind to wander. Make sure you have some food and water. Alcohol, drugs, and junk food are completely off limits. Eat real food only. If you want to spend some of the time cooking a delicious meal, great—just make sure it's *real food.*

One final rule about this: Do not just sleep or lie in bed the whole time. It would be great if you could get out and take a walk in nature, get a hotel room by yourself for the day, go for a bike ride, or go kayaking—whatever you can do without bumping into too many people who might try to talk with you. You can wave hello and nod your head to acknowledge someone, but stay in silence.

You can do this anywhere—even in NYC. A big city is a great place to do this, in fact, because it is highly unlikely that you will bump into someone you know. And even if you do, *bam!* Whip out your note!

Your most important task during these twenty-four hours is to be completely bored. You want to be so bored that you *have to have* a few conversations with yourself while staring at the tree outside your window or watching the crack in the paint in the corner of the room. Let that boredom turn into peace, and use this time to reconnect with yourself. You'll learn that when you really let your mind wander—when it's truly *just you* and your inner thoughts, your innate intelligence—you get reconnected, and you start to make a connection with the person who matters the most: *You!*

> **RULE:**
>
> Reconnect with yourself. Spend at least twenty-four hours with *just you.*

Journaling

I've already shared my feelings about journaling, but it's such a fantastic exercise that I'll briefly mention it again here. Everyone should make it part of their life on a regular basis. I've been on "journaling weekends," events where we just hike and talk and think, then sit for an hour and journal our thoughts—that's something completely different, and you might want to try something like that to help you increase your grade in *Connectedness.*

The process I described in the chapter about stress is for quick journaling throughout the day to help you connect, clear your mind, or relax and sleep by getting the immediate thoughts out of your head. I would highly recommend doing this at any time throughout the day to help you connect with yourself more, but, at the very least, do it before bed so you can have the most restful sleep possible.

Meditation

Boy, am I happy I'm not writing a book on meditation! The subject of meditation could be discussed indefinitely. I'm just going to give you some brief tips for how to set up some meditation rules for yourself.

What do you need to know about meditation? First, I believe meditation is a incredibly helpful tool for managing stress and reconnecting with yourself and your innate intelligence. Meditation is essential for me. It doesn't replace eating right, exercising, or having a great relationship with close family and friends, but you could also argue that all these other habits come much more easily to one who meditates on a regular basis. Whatever way you choose to implement this rule—whether first or last—it must be done. So, let's go through some basics on how to do meditate.

Meditation might sound intimidating, but it doesn't have to be difficult. There are countless ways to meditate, and it doesn't have to take much time. You can meditate for a few minutes, for hours ... or even days on end. Whatever you choose is up to you. Personally, I meditate to slow down my racing brain and as a way to reconnect daily with my innate self.

Meditation can be as simple as taking a few seconds here and there throughout your day to recognize that you are an amazing, living, breathing, wondrous being. Take a couple seconds right now—put down this book for a moment—and take seven breaths in through your nose and out your mouth. Try to recognize your heartbeat during those breaths ... feel the air going into and out of your lungs ... feel your chest expanding and contracting... .

I'll wait... .

... Are you done? Great.

Meditating can start off as simple as that. It's about being "in the now," as Eckhart Tolle says. In order to get the most out of meditation, I think you should read a book or two or take a few classes about Buddhism. Learn more—you can get to the mastery level if you like, but just starting somewhere and making meditation a part of your life is immensely rewarding.

Here are a few ways that I meditate. Some are less conventional than others, but I get that same "connected" feeling from them all. For me, it's about the sense of connectedness that I've been talking about: connectedness with myself, God, the universe, and my innate intelligence. It feels good and creates a release of many positive chemicals and endorphins in my body.

You have the ability to create all the chemicals you need to feel great right now, already inside of you. At least, you have the *potential* to reconnect yourself. Once you do experience the feeling of innate connectedness, there is no other feeling like it except love.

Here are some tools I teach and use that will help you get connected!

Four-Seven-Eight

This is an easy breathing and centering technique I picked up while watching Dr. Andrew Weil about twenty years ago. It's so simple and effective that I've used it ever since.

- Place the tip of your tongue behind your two top front teeth. (This is third eye stimulation, supposedly. I don't question; it can't hurt, so I just do it).
- Take a deep breath in through your nose for a count of four.
- Hold your breath for a count of seven.
- Breathe out slowly through your mouth for a count of eight (because your tongue is behind your teeth, you will end up making a hissing sound as you exhale).
- Repeat seven times.

That's it! Four-seven-eight, seven times. If you're feeling anxious, your mind is racing, or you can't relax, it's a great tool to control your breathing and your mind. You see, you can't think of many other things while you're doing this exercise—you're too busy counting. The fact that you're controlling your breathing is also beneficial. One thing we tend to lose control of when we are caught up in daily life is our ability to properly take a deep breath and get more oxygen to our brains. This exercise takes care of both things: It's a distraction mentally, and it allows you to take control of your body for a couple minutes, reset your nervous system, and get you more connected.

Forty-Nine Breaths

Need more energy? Need to focus? Want to start your day with inspiration? Forty-nine breaths is the way to go. Forty-nine breaths, as far as I know, is an old chiropractic method of meditating, created by (or at least popularized by) Dr. Sid Williams, one of the greatest healers and champions of health this earth has ever known. Here's how to do it.

- Sit up straight on a stool or bench, or, if your chair has a back to it, scoot forward toward the end.
- You should be barefoot and wearing comfortable clothes.
- Place your palms face down on your knees.
- Take seven deep breaths in through your nose and out through your mouth, each being very deep and powerful breaths. You need to relax your belly for this so you can take a nice deep breath through your abdomen, then use your diaphragm to push the air out. The breathing should be rather vigorous. It may even give you a buzz at first from being lightheaded.
- After the first seven breaths, place your palms face up, take a nice long breath in, and let out a sweeping sigh.
- Now, begin to say some positive affirmations. Let your mind go ... tell yourself how healthy and happy you are. Tell yourself how great a mother you are, how amazing a father you are, what a great person you are, how in love with life you are, what you have accomplished. (An accomplishment might also be a current goal of yours, but you should envision it as if it has already happened). You get the picture.
- When you feel like you've said enough (ten seconds to two minutes), put your palms face down again on your knees and take fourteen big breaths in through your nose and out through your mouth.
- Take another long breath and a sweeping sigh.
- Palms up again and say some more affirmations—ten seconds to two minutes.
- Repeat the fourteen breaths/sighs/affirmations two more times, and you will hit forty-nine breaths!
- As a bonus, when you're done, belt out a few *Oms*.
- *Om... .*

- Give it all you've got until you run out of breath, and then do it again!

Sample positive affirmations to start you off:

- I feel *healthy*
- I feel *happy*
- I feel *terrific*
- I am at peace
- I am love
- I am happiness
- I am joy
- I am grateful

- I am a great healer
- I am a great listener
- I am a great husband
- I am a great father
- I love what I do
- I love who I am
- I am success
- I am one with God

You get the picture?

You can get as detailed as you want:

- I have created and I am still creating the life of my dreams!
- I am filled with happiness, joy, and love!
- I give of myself every day, and the universe has granted me the wisdom and unique ability to share my abundant life with all of those who are ready to receive abundance around me.

Classic Meditation:

The basic premise behind most of the classic forms of meditation I have learned over the course of a decade of meditation practice comes down to this:

FOCUS ON ONE THOUGHT FOR AS LONG AS YOU CAN

That's it! There are classes, books, websites, gurus, weeklong retreats ... all focused on helping you to do one simple thing. Focus on one thought, one image, one mantra, your breath, as long as you can. And when you realize that your mind has wandered off and started thinking about another thing—or dozens of other things—reset your focus back to the thing you were focusing on in the first place.

It's crazy how simple it is, yet I have spent countless hours practicing and learning about meditation, and I still feel like I absolutely suck at it. Yet I keep doing it! I have a daily practice of meditation because it helps me. For some of you, meditation will simply become calming your seventy thoughts down to ten. For others, you will get "lost" in your mantra. There are many levels in between. I feel like I've experienced them all.

Keep in mind that meditation is called a *practice*. There isn't necessarily some end goal to reach. The practice of meditation is like an exercise for your mind. This exercise works on gaining control over what is called the "monkey mind." It is the state when we close our eyes and we can't control the thoughts. Practicing meditation gets you to work on it so you can be *better* at it. I hope you get so good at it that you will obtain enlightenment! I haven't yet, but I will keep practicing.

I will give you a list of my favorite resources for meditation so you can find out more and begin your practice. They are listed at the end of the book as well.

- Mindvalleyacademy.com (my favorite is the Silva life System but there are so many great resources)
- pemachodronfoundation.org
- audiodharma.org
- Apps: Headspace and Calm
- Intro to meditation: *10% Happier* by Dan Harris

RULE:

If you haven't been practicing meditation, begin as soon as possible!

Listen to Others

You can do guided meditations as well. There are plenty of CDs, internet links, and videos out there. Some of the ones I mentioned before have great guided meditations. Find one that you enjoy and that clicks with you. Listen to it and learn your own way to meditate!

Exercise as Meditation

When I first started meditating, there were times when I felt I wasn't ready for it. There were times I couldn't get my mind to stop racing. Either that or I would just fall asleep. The form of meditation that I used during that stage of my life (and that I still use today) was long, monotonous, challenging cardiovascular exercise. I either used cycling (especially good if you are climbing up hills), jogging, and hiking.

You can use whatever you like—just don't bring that iPod or MP3 player with you! For meditation, you need to be alone with your thoughts. If you're exercising at a pace that is at least mildly challenging, you can get into a zone where all you can think of is getting to a certain point: up that next ridge ... to that stop sign ... past that rock... . Then you can pick a new point. Maintain your focus on something simple. Sometimes, when I'm riding my bike up a hill, all I do in my head is repeat the *Rocky* theme song over and over again. If you feel like quiet meditation is too much at the beginning, you can still get to that great state of connectedness by doing physical activity like this. It's not as peaceful as still meditation, but it's a beneficial practice and a great way to get started.

> **RULE:**
>
> When you feel your mind is racing and you simply cannot sit and close your eyes and meditate, try a twenty-minute walk where you are mindful of your surroundings and your breath and nothing else!

Chapter 18

Health Awareness

The "space between our ears" is one of the most significant contributors to our quality of life. Thoughts are *things*. Our thoughts are extremely real, and when we become stuck in self-limiting beliefs, it becomes challenging for us to find solutions for the issues we face. It also becomes challenging to keep improving our grades in all of the areas of our personal report cards.

Health awareness is, in part, about knowing what to do to improve your marks and your overall HPA. As you become more aware of how important each of the areas on your report card is, and how important it is to have a high grade in each for your overall quality of life, you will be on your way to improvement.

Health awareness is about educating yourself about healthy topics on a regular basis. It's great that you've made the effort to read this book, but there is so much more out there. The only reason I live the life I do and keep the habits I keep is that every day, I read at least a little something new that reminds me *why* I'm doing it. I read articles, listen to TED Talks, read more books, go to lectures... . I'm not suggesting you need to do as much as I do. It's my job to stay informed so I can teach you about health, but you can't rely on one book or one article to keep you on track. If you want a great place to enhance your grade, simply follow me on Facebook and or Twitter. I post articles, videos, book recommendations, and anything I'm truly excited about and I think would improve your *Health Awareness* grade.

@drpiken

www.facebook.com/innatechiromanhattan/

My favorite quote to use when it comes to many habits—but especially health awareness—is "the mind always wants more" by Maharishi Mahesh Yogi. When I first heard this simple statement, it hit me as some of the most profound words I had ever heard. That short phrase sums up how our minds function and what drives us to do what we do each day. I'll elaborate. If you expose your mind to stressful or negative information each day, you will tend to see the world as stressful and negative. If you expose yourself to peaceful, uplifting, and positive information, then you will tend to see the world differently.

Let's use some real-life examples that I have seen over the years. The first example is Marci. Marci grew up in a lower-middle-class home where her family always struggled to make ends meet. She was taught "keep your head down and work hard because life isn't easy." Marci has lived within the same fifteen-mile radius her whole life and hasn't traveled much. Marci's daily routine begins with waking up, turning on the news, and listening to what is happening so she can be "better informed" about her day. Marci eats a lot of starchy foods. She just started eating salads, but she puts gobs of salad dressing on top for flavor. Marci is an avid reader. She tends to read romance novels and suspenseful thrillers; she also has a weakness for celebrity gossip magazines. Can you guess what type of grades Marci gets on her report card?

Marci's world is shaped by what she exposes her mind to every day. Marci was first exposed to what life is about by her family, who had learned it from previous generations. Marci begins her day with the local news. When you begin your day learning about all of the local murders, accidents, school shootings, wars, and businesses that were "caught doing wrong," it shapes your view of the world. To "escape," she reads about fantasy. She doesn't believe that any of the amazing things that happen to the characters in her romance novels will come true for her. Marci believes that most people simply suck! Wouldn't you, if you watched the housewives shows every day? I think you can get the picture by now. Marci's views of the world have been and continue to be shaped by what she *chooses* to expose her mind to each and every day.

I tried educating Marci for years. I recommended new types of books, told her to stop watching the news in the morning, taught her why nourishing foods were essential. I worked very hard at reprogramming her brain by getting her to change her habits. But, in the end, she never followed through with the recommendations I suggested. She had a fixed mindset. She didn't believe she could change who she was, so she never even tried. Have you ever heard the Henry Ford quote, "Whether you think you can or you think you can't—you're right"?

Health awareness is also about the art of self-reflection and being aware of your thoughts and beliefs. Which beliefs do you currently hold that are limiting you? If you walk around every day with the belief that you're never going to improve your grade in *Exercise*, for example, it's going to be difficult to be motivated enough to take the actions necessary *to actually improve your grade.* Health awareness enables you to assess your beliefs and discard those that are no longer serving you.

Let's now contrast Marci's story with Benjy's story. Benjy had a very similar upbringing. He had a lot of similar habits, as well. Benjy came to me with complaints of neck pain. Like most people, he thought he would go the chiropractor for a "crack" to get his neck to feel better. Benjy was in for a surprise. On each patient's second visit, I give them a report. During this report, I discuss everything I believe to be the cause of their problems. During Benjy's report, I shared that I believed his pain was coming from the fact that he needs to improve his lifestyle, not because he needed a "crack" in his back.

Benjy is one of those patients I dream of filling my practice with. His eyes lit up with excitement. He asked me why no one had ever explained these things to him. Benjy began to change his life bit by bit. He stopped watching the news in the morning, he put better things into his body, he began to exercise, and he began reading about health-related topics. He altered what his mind was exposed to every day.

Can you guess where Marci and Benjy are today? To be honest, I'm not sure about Marci. When someone doesn't follow through with the recommendations I prescribe, it's only a matter of time before I stop seeing them as a patient. Meanwhile, Benjy has transformed from an overweight, slouched-postured, chronically pain-ridden young man into a competitive triathlete. Sure, Benjy still has aches and pains. His grades still aren't straight As. He's made small changes over many years because he did the most import-ant thing first. He decided to learn about healthy living and spend time exposing his mind to new ideas on a reg-ular basis.

A great way to keep your thoughts and mindset in a good place is to feed your brain with positive messages on a regular basis. For example, listen to a podcast on your way to work. As I mentioned in Part III, I make listening to a podcast part of my morning routine.

Reading books written by people you consider mentors or whose information uplifts you is also a good way to improve your mindset. The most important element in terms of keeping a good mindset is regularly feeding your mind with things that empower you and help you create beliefs that inspire you. What you input is what you will output—meaning, if you feed your mind great things, you will think great thoughts and bring those great thoughts into your day, making great things happen. And even if you're faced with a challenge, when you have the right mindset, you can move through the challenge and see solutions much more easily. Your mindset is like the context for your day—the filter through which you see everything that happens during your day.

A positive mindset helps you be more health-aware. One of the main tenets of personal development and inspirational books or podcasts is that you have the ability to affect something in your life given *the way you think about it and what you believe to be true about it.* And, in general, working on your mindset is the natural action to take as you become more and more health-aware because the health-aware individual understands the importance of tending to the garden of their mind.

In addition to working on your mindset, improve your health awareness by always looking for ways you can improve in all of the areas on your report card. Have you gone through a couple of report card assessments and gotten the highest grades possible in an area? Change your grading scheme to push you toward getting even better in that area.

Have you consistently declined in one area because the grading scheme is over your head and demoralizing you? Make the adjustments required to make it the right tool to push you toward improvement. Do you need to add in a few more rules for yourself or create a ritual as part of your day?

Life is fluid, as is improvement. As you use your report card, keep looking at yourself and seeing what you need to change to keep getting better in every area.

RULE:

Follow @Drpiken on Twitter and "like" Innate Chiropractic of Manhattan on Facebook—I only post articles, audios, and videos that will increase your grade in *Health Awareness*!

Chapter 19

Elimination

*E*limination is a big indicator of your *Diet* grade. Believe it or not, you'd be amazed at what your poop reveals about your health—and your HPA! When I learn that a patient of mine has any type of irregularity in their bowel movements—whether in the frequency and or in the quality of their poop—I want to understand why.

The health of your poop is, in part, a reflection of the health of your digestive system. Why should you pay attention to that? Well, the number-one reason for me is that your immune system, your ability to fight infections, cancer, and your ability to heal, is intimately tied to the health of your gut! Need I say more?

Irregular Bowel Movements—Not Enough or Too Hard

Are you saying to yourself, "I'm not going to the bathroom enough?" My definition of "not enough" movements is having less than one bowel movement per day or feeling like you don't evacuate completely *each time*. I reiterate the same information about any chronic ailment: chronic, recurring, or even occasional irregularity *is* a problem that should be addressed. The vast majority of the time, the problem is solved by changing and improving your habits.

Improving your bowel movements may be addressed by following four simple rules: Get enough fiber in your diet, drink enough water, have enough friendly microorganisms living in and on your body, and ingest enough magnesium. If you follow these rules, most irregularities will go away. Let's address them one by one.

1. Fiber

Based on a study published in the journal *Advances in Nutrition*, the average adult male should be ingesting 38 grams of fiber per day. The average female should be ingesting 25 grams of fiber per day.[5]

If you want to know why we should ingest at least the recommended daily intake of fiber, Google "the benefits of fiber," and you will learn about it. Fiber must be part of your daily life, and you should prioritize it in your habits. To figure out how to improve your fiber intake so you can reach your fiber goals, use the following simple exercise.

Write down the food you eat in a typical twenty-four hours and approximate the portions. Then Google the words "fiber chart." You'll see a few sites pop up that list foods and the amount of fiber per serving of those foods. Now, just do the math and add up the fiber in your day. If you are far from your target number, you now can see how to increase fiber in your diet by using the list of foods in the fiber chart. Keep in mind that you should do this gradually—if you increase from a diet of 10 grams of fiber a day to 35 grams of fiber per day *overnight*, you will probably become bloated, uncomfortable, and even angry. Increase your fiber by 3 to 4 grams per day every few days.

If you have any challenges with the way you feel with this increase in diet, make sure you work with a knowledgeable health practitioner to guide you through the process.

2. Water

We need to have enough water in our systems in order to have healthy stools. My general rule, as I mentioned in the *Hydration* chapter, Chapter 13, is to drink half your body weight in fluid ounces per day. If this sounds like a lot, make it a goal that you build up to gradually. As a side effect of drinking more water, you will also tend to eat less because you're hydrated and filled with water. Review the chapter on hydration to learn more.

3. Microorganisms

I talk about microorganisms and the microbiome in more detail in the upcoming chapter, "Special Circumstances." For now, I'll give a brief summary: We all have little bugs inside us that help us digest our foods and are a part of our immune systems. There are "friendly bugs" that help us and "unfriendly bugs" that don't and can cause discomfort and unhappiness. These bugs can shift and change based on factors such as what we are eating and drinking, our stress levels, medications we take, old infections, and other variables.

If you begin to eat the way you are supposed to eat, there will be a gradual increase in the number of "good bugs" compared to "bad bugs." One very important fact that we should all know is that humans cannot digest fiber. We need these friendly bugs to break down the undigested fiber in our digestive tract and to help us form a healthy bowel movement. You can increase the "good bugs" by eating more fiber, eating fermented foods like sauerkraut, kimchi, and Kombucha, and by taking the right kind of probiotic supplements. A lot of people have heard of probiotic strains; Acidophilus is a well-known one. There are many different kinds of good bacteria, and one that works for one person may not be the same one that works for another. I usually start patients on a supplement made by Metagenics called *Ultraflora Balance* to test the waters. It's a blend of "good bugs" commonly found in the adult gut. Again, for more info, I have a whole chapter on this coming up called Special Circumstances.

4. Magnesium

This is the last but equally important ingredient that we need for healthy poop. We all need magnesium in our diets, and based on my observations in treating thousands of patients over the years, I have found that virtually *no one* is getting enough in their diets. Foods that contain high amounts of magnesium include:

- Dark, leafy, green veggies (e.g., kale, spinach, broccoli... .)
- Fish
- Nuts and seeds
- Beans and lentils
- Avocados
- Bananas
- Start by increasing magnesium-rich foods in your diet, and if that doesn't help after a couple of weeks, get a magnesium supplement. I use a few different types in my office, so I don't want to recommend a specific brand in this book. From my experience, it seems that different forms of magnesium work best for different types of individuals. While experimenting, keep in mind the same recommendations I shared for introducing fiber. It's important to *gradually* introduce magnesium into your life as a supplement. If you take too much, it will cause loose stool and could cause some bloating as well.

If you consult with a professional who understands how to recommend it properly, you can learn more about which type is right for you and how to take it.

Irregular Bowel Movements—Too Frequent or Loose Stool

Here are my recommendations to people that have loose or overly frequent bowel movements. First things first: *find out why!* There's often a pattern. Maybe you have loose stool every time you eat spicy foods or drink alcohol or eat pasta or eat too many French fries or ... get the picture? If you already know that certain foods cause your poop to be loose, then *stop it!* Stop eating foods that bother you! What are you? Stupid? Of course you are—so am I! At times, I do things that my body doesn't like, but as I get older, learn, and understand more, I do those stupid things less often. So the first rule is to stop knowingly hurting yourself with the things you put in your body.

The next thing to ask yourself is, "How am I handling stress?" If you think your diet is great but you're under a lot of stress, that can impact the quality of your bowel movements as well. Go right to the section on *Stress Management* and begin to raise your grade!

Still don't know why your bowel movements are too frequent or too loose? If you feel that your stress is low and well managed and your diet is amazing, then the next thing I would recommend is to consult a qualified health practitioner to help figure this out. There are parasites, worms, and many subtle food allergies and sensitivities that can also cause loose stool, and it's a good idea to rule these out as the cause for your symptoms.

If after implementing these rules you're still not pooping properly, then you may need to visit a qualified health professional. Sometimes, a medical doctor can help, but keep in mind that most of the time they will prescribe a medication that might make you poop but won't necessarily make you *healthier*. That doesn't make sense to me. I would recommend finding a naturopath, a chiropractor, a nutritionist, or an acupuncturist—someone who understands how to get you healthy. But try these solutions first. I think you'll find they are enough to help you raise your grade in this area!

> **RULE:**
>
> To stay regular and have a healthy elimination process, follow the four rules for healthy elimination: fiber, water, microorganisms, and magnesium.

PART V
Keeping Your Grades Up

Chapter 20

Special Circumstances

A t least 80 percent of the time I work with patients, there are some very simple rules that, if followed, will create abundant health. But the other 20 percent of the time, there are more complicated cases that, unfortunately, are beginning to encompass a larger percentage of my practice. These people have followed the "rules," and they haven't gotten results. Food sensitivities, toxins, and leaky gut syndrome are some of the common reasons.

This Special Circumstances chapter is meant to address the concerns of anyone experiencing these specific issues or diagnoses that directly affect health and quality of life. This covers some of the most common issues I see patients dealing with that prevent them from making progress in their journey towards healthy lives.

People often get frustrated when their underlying health issues aren't being resolved. If they don't feel better, they take breaks from or even abandon their health goals altogether. I mentioned in earlier chapters that I am seeing an increasing percentage of patients who deal with more complicated symptoms. What works for most people simply doesn't work for others, even when they follow the same rules. These patients have typically been to multiple doctors before they find their way to my office. They have been told things like: "It's all in your head," or "There's nothing you can do, so you'll just have to live with it." These people have had MRIs. They've had multiple lab tests. They've tried many medications. But they still don't feel that their issues are being addressed.

Unfortunately, that's when these people finally find me: as a last resort. I'm not their first choice for their health-care needs, as I would prefer. The longer someone has been living with their symptoms—or worse, ignoring them—the more challenging it is to work with them. This isn't because they are incurable; it's usually because they find it hard to grasp the idea that they need to put in the weeks or months required to allow their bodies enough time to heal from years of poor habits and lifestyle. The body has an incredible ability to heal, yet one of those magic ingredients necessary for the healing process is *time*.

There is a principle in chiropractic from the original *Chiropractic Text Book* by R.W. Stephenson that states simply, "There is no process that does not require time." That principle works in two ways: It takes time to cause your problems, and it also takes time, once you begin the healing process, to achieve results. One of the main reasons I focus on teaching healthy living rather than merely removing symptoms is because by focusing on how you feel every day, you will inevitably get frustrated with the real process of healing. Sure, it's great to feel good, and most of my patients' symptoms do alleviate when I work with them, *but* the patients who achieve the greatest results also understand that the care that we give is different than most other healthcare offices. I ask them to take an active part in changing their lives, and the ones who dive in, make those changes, and give the process time to take hold always get the best results.

The following pages outline some of the more stubborn, challenging, gray areas of health that I work with. I say "gray areas" because sometimes there is no specific diagnosis for these issues. These are not diseases that can be treated; these are symptoms. These are issues that many people are chronically dealing with that keep them from feeling better as quickly as they would like. My job is to work with my patients throughout the process of figuring out the unique, individual circumstances that have been holding them back

In the following pages, I'll discuss a few common special circumstances so that you have some general advice regarding each of these things, should they come up for you at any time.

Toxicity

Toxins from our environment are affecting us all in some way, shape, or form. This is because we encounter so many toxins in our environment on a daily basis. These days, we find toxins in our food, our water, and our air. Over time, toxins can build up and start to overwhelm the bodies and our immune systems.

What is a toxin? Simply put, a toxin is anything that gets into our body and is recognized as foreign. Your body reacts to toxins appropriately, attacking them as an invader that should be fought and removed. It's similar to the reaction your body has when combatting a virus. The body should recognize the invader and try to make sure it doesn't hurt you. So the more toxins you are exposed to, the more likely your immune system—and your detoxification system—will be overburdened. When it's overburdened, it may start to decrease its function, or it may shift into "overdrive" (this is similar to what happens with sensitivities and intolerances to food, discussed in the next section).

How did we become so toxic? Let's go back to the early 1800s. At the beginning of the American Industrial

Revolution, we were surely exposed to more toxins than ever before in human history. The toxins were substances that humans had been exposed to throughout history, but during the Industrial Revolution, we became exposed to them in a much more concentrated fashion. There were massive factories and sweatshops. People worked with giant machines that spit out toxins, and at the time, we didn't understand how the byproducts of all this production were affecting us.

Unfortunately, even after big companies learned about the harm they are causing, they didn't always rectify the problem. After many years of scientific discovery and understanding—many years of illness, suffering, and protests for change—working conditions slowly improved. Clean air and sanitation standards were implemented, which improved working conditions by keeping the toxin exposure at "acceptable" levels. But really, there isn't any "acceptable" level of mercury, aluminum, arsenic, coal, or soot in the human body; we have merely come to *accept* that a small amount will only harm a small amount of people.

I don't want to go back to the times before machines—I like modern living—but all this innovation comes at a price. We've created so many new chemicals, some of them originating from "natural" sources, but those "natural" compounds are so concentrated that they can become lethal. Think of something as simple as aspirin. Aspirin, or acetylsalicylic acid, comes from tree bark. Yet if you extract a small component from this natural source and ingest too much of it, you could die. If you take even small amounts on a regular basis, you can irritate the lining of your intestines and burden your liver.

We may find positive uses for concentrated substances in our lives, but it usually comes at the expense of some type of side effect. So we find "acceptable levels" for these "natural" concentrates. The standard is usually the amount that will help us without screwing up too many people. But no matter what, some people are still affected negatively. And these days, that number is on the rise as these toxins and chemicals build up in our bodies.

Now, in 2016, we have thousands of "natural" and artificial chemicals that we are exposed to every single day. Soot on our window sills, dry cleaning chemicals, chemical food additives, pesticides, plastics ... we can go on listing them forever! These chemicals are allowed to be expelled into the environment because they have received a GRAS or "Generally Regarded As Safe" rating. What that means is that studies have been done—rarely human studies—regarding these chemicals. The researchers determine that exposure to this chemical in higher than usual amounts won't *likely* kill us or *probably* won't cause cancer.

What nobody is addressing, however, is the combination of all of the toxins we're exposed to and how they *interplay* with each other and affect the human body. That has never been studied because it's *impossible* to do so. There are thousands of chemicals we're exposed to now that we were not exposed to 200 years ago. There is simply no way to test for all of the combinations of these chemicals or how they affect us.

What does all of this do to your wonderful immune system and liver? If your body is constantly battling foreign objects, it can get overloaded and malfunction. Also, every person has a different tolerance for the toxins we're exposed to. How do you feel after drinking a beer? How about six beers? How about twelve? I'm sure we all know that everyone handles alcohol differently. One person can get drunk after a single drink, and another is able to handle much more, sometimes for no apparent reason.

We can't avoid toxins. Instead, the key is to get rid of them as quickly as they enter our bodies. How do you do this? One way is to learn about the toxins in our environment. We should all be educated about where these toxins come from. Another way is to *detox*! Get rid of the chemicals you've been exposed to over the course of, literally, your whole life.

First, how can you tell if you're toxic? The answer isn't so simple. The symptoms of a toxic, overburdened body are vague. Some of the common symptoms of a toxic body are actually some of the most common complaints that people ignore or "learn to live with" every day. Aches and pains—headaches and muscle or joint aches. There are other symptoms as well, such as dizziness, trouble losing weight, brain fog, and fatigue. Toxicity and an overactive immune system can turn into even more severe developments and can interfere with your ability to heal.

Detoxing *can* make you better. The whole point of detoxing is to decrease your exposure to chemicals and give your body space to heal. As a positive side effect as well, detoxing will likely set in place the changes you need to boost your grade in *Diet*!

Leaky Gut

One of the ways chemicals can enter your body is because of a condition called "leaky gut." One of the leading ways a toxin enters our body is when we eat it! We're either eating it, smelling it, or it's being absorbed through our skin. The following is my simple leaky gut story.

It starts when we eat something that we're not supposed to eat, like pesticide residue, food coloring, a food we're sensitive to, or maybe just massive amounts of hot sauce. Whatever it is, it's just not supposed to be inside your body.

When you first ingest something, it isn't technically inside your body yet. It's just passing through this tube known as your digestive tract. That tube starts in your mouth and ends at your anus. Until you absorb the substance that you placed in your mouth, it's just passing through. The way a substance enters your body is through a process called active transport. Simply put, our innate intelligence is supposed to pick and choose the digested ingredients it needs to support us and reject the ingredients it doesn't. Think of your digestive tract as rubber hose that has the ability to let beneficial nutrients leak through the wall of the hose but will allow less beneficial substances or toxins to keep moving all the way through to the other end. If we keep exposing this tube to too many toxins, the barrier system gets worn down, and more toxins enter the body. Fortunately, we have these great organs in our body to help out when this happens.

Your liver and kidneys help you to recognize and eliminate toxins that mistakenly get absorbed. Remember from the beginning of the book, though, the very important statement I mentioned: Symptoms are caused by the accumulation of stress! If we burden our bodies for years, our ability to handle this chemical stress can be overwhelmed. Your gut can become irritated by these toxins and by eating foods you're not supposed to be eating.

Let's say you eat junk food your whole life—more than you can handle. The barrier between the outside world, which is more toxic, and our inside body, which shouldn't be toxic, gets broken down. Our intestinal wall should prevent the absorption of these toxins, but, it gets worn out. That's what we call leaky gut.

So, how do you prevent leaky gut? Start by eating clean, unadulterated food. Some foods that are good to eat for a healthy detox are cruciferous vegetables, which consists of the cabbage family of vegetables. They contain phyto-nutrients like glucosinolates, which can help the immune system. Limonene is a great phytonutrient that's also found in citrus fruits. Sulfur foods like eggs are also great. Eggs were vilified for decades because of a mistaken claim about cholesterol. Research has refuted this evidence, having now shown for many years that eggs have little to no effect on cholesterol. Eggs are one of the most perfect foods on the planet, unless you're sensitive to them—some people are. In that case, you'll want to limit your intake. But, in general, eggs are very healthy.

Cumin and turmeric are also great for regulating the in-flammatory response in the body. Keeping down inflamma-tion helps the detox process. Cinnamon, onion, and garlic are natural antibacterial agents and help the body to detox, as long as you're not sensitive to them. Milk thistle is an herb famous for aiding in detox—it supports your liver. Ar-tichoke leaf is also great.

Certain supplements also support a healthy detox. Start with B vitamins at first. B vitamins are pretty easy to with-draw from food. They're found in whole grains, cruciferous vegetables, and leafy greens. Given the way we eat and the way our food is processed today, it's becoming harder and harder to get enough B vitamins from food alone. We might get enough to survive, but we don't take supplements to survive; we take them to *thrive*. We also need more vita-mins when our body is burdened by the chemicals in our environment.

In terms of actual cleanse/detox programs, there are a lot out there. I can't keep track of every single product, so I don't recommend any type of product other than those I work with. Others could also be great. What you have to watch out for when picking a cleanse/detox program is that it doesn't just make you poop your brains out without offering any real nutrition. Also, watch out for programs from companies that don't do strict testing. Just because a supplement has a stamp on the bottle that states how great the company is, it doesn't mean the stamp is valid in the first place.

Some of the most common products I use for enhancing people's bodies via cleansing and detoxing are Metagenics UltraInflamX, Clearvite from Apex Energetics, and the Six-day Detox kit from Xymogen. I trust where they come from. I've personally been taking Metagenics UltraInflamX three to four times a week for about fourteen years. Do your research or get advice from a trusted source about which cleanse/detox program to try. How you use the program needs to be individually based. Sure, there are protocols, so talk to a trusted source to reach the next level of clearance.

If your toxicity levels are high, the most important thing to do is to clean out your system to prevent the external and internal toxins from building up, triggering your immune system to go out of control. There are too many toxins in our environment these days and too few detoxifiers in our food supply. Take in more detoxifying foods, supplements, and herbs. Make sure to enhance detoxification pathways in your body so you can combat the toxic load taken on in modern life.

Food Sensitivities and Intolerances

First, let's state that food sensitivities and intolerances are different than food allergies. Explaining the differences between food allergies and sensitivities goes beyond the scope of this book. I want you to use this book to learn the basics. This section is only meant to raise awareness about sensitivities and intolerances.

Food sensitivities and intolerances are more common than most people think. The issue with them is that exposure to sensitivities contributes to inflammation in our bodies—one of the two *whys* from the beginning of this book.

To understand the basics of food sensitivities, you have to understand how the immune system works in general. When your body encounters a pathogen (a virus, a type of bacteria, or a parasite) the body attacks it. Pathogens are *not* symbiotic. They don't work *with* us. They just want to reproduce—it's the only thing they do. A pathogen wants to thrive and reproduce and live off of us, essentially, and the body does its best to circumvent this. The immune system recognizes when something bad enters the body and fights it. In the case of food sensitivities and intolerances, the body thinks that a certain food itself is a pathogen and turns the immune response up to "fight" it. This puts unnecessary stress on the immune system.

Food sensitivities/allergies have probably been around forever, but they're a lot more prevalent now than they've ever been before. There are many reasons why. Toxins and leaky gut can allow food particles into our bodies that are either larger than they should be or are bound to chemicals. If your body sets up an immune response to this food particle, even a single time, it recognizes that food as an enemy and will keep targeting it for the rest of your life, attacking that food every time it invades the body.

If you keep exposing your body to this food over and over again, you can become even more sensitive to it. Gluten, discussed in Chapter 6, is a prime example. Most of us have eaten gluten for decades in its many forms, since wheat products are found in so many processed foods. After developing a sensitivity and having years of exposure, your body can develop even stronger immune reactions. You could have eaten a food your entire life and *suddenly* feel the effects of a sensitivity to this food in your twenties, thirties, or even sixties. If you eat an ingredient on a regular basis and it causes your immune system to react, that reaction can become more severe as years go by. This is why we can develop food sensitivities after years of eating foods that we felt fine with in the past.

The quality of our food has also gotten poorer throughout the ages. Food is not *food*, at least not in this country. Virtually everything is covered in pesticides or has antibiotics or hormones in it. Even if you're eating organic, our soils have been contaminated, and our air is contaminated. There is very little pure, clean food anymore, especially on our continent. Often, patients with multiple food sensitivities find that when they travel around the world, they can eat whatever they want and feel fine.

Food sensitivities and intolerances become more of a problem the more toxins you put into your body. Often someone is mildly sensitive, and then a trauma, an inflammatory injury, or surgery will trigger a more severe reaction. A good detox/cleanse is usually needed to help heal the overactive inflammatory response. This helps to take the load off your body and encourages it to start functioning normally again.

You *can* heal your immune system and start feeling better. How long does it take? It's different for everybody. You just have to give yourself time to heal. It depends on how resilient you are and how long the issues have existed.

There is also a common diet I recommend. Many people don't want to take a lot of vitamins and herbs, so we begin by simply changing their diet to try to figure out which foods are affecting them and how. The program I use most often in my practice evaluates and helps people to heal from food sensitivities and intolerances is a version of the autoimmune (or AI) paleo diet.

I'll give you a brief background. The foods at the beginning of the diet are foods that humans have been eating since the beginning. Meats, fats, vegetables, and fruit. They also tend to be the foods that the fewest number of people are sensitive to. You might be sensitive to something in the beginning of the plan, but if you are, it is likely that your digestive system needs to be cleansed by a specific program. You should work with your health practitioner first.

Begin the program with a strict, limited diet. After a predetermined number of weeks (two for the generally healthy and up to twelve for highly sensitive people of those with chronic issues or autoimmune diseases), you slowly reintroduce foods that you have been avoiding. That is, as long as you were feeling better in the first step of the process, of course.

The vast majority of people who follow this plan do feel better. Less bloated, more energy, fewer aches and pains—these are a few of the more common reactions to the initial stage. As you reintroduce foods, one new group each week, try to sense if there are any differences in the way you feel. If you begin to eat something that you are sensitive or allergic to, you might experience a symptom within twelve to twenty-four hours, or it could even take up to a week. The goal is to learn how eating different foods affects how you feel.

Please keep in mind that although you are technically allowed to eat as much meat and fat as you want, the best thing to do is to follow some of the earlier recommendations from the *Diet* section and eat small, frequent meals consisting of 70 percent vegetables. There is a website that does the best job at explaining the ins and outs of the autoimmune paleo diet: autoimmunewellness.com./ I have created a quick reference/cheat sheet that I use with my patients as well. Here is my quick reference sheet:

1. Restricted Paleo Diet
Eat only:
• Meats, seafood, poultry: best wild or grass-fed, organic, not fed grains or soy

- Fats: olive oil, coconut oil, avocados, lard, bacon fat, cultured ghee (certified to be free of casein and lactose)
- All fruits and veggies with the exception of nightshades: best starch—sweet potato
- Raw honey

2. After two to twelve weeks (dependent on individual needs), reintroduce in order. Allow one week between any new foods introduced and note reactions you may have to the reintroduced foods.

- Nuts and seeds (keep in mind that peanuts are not nuts; they are legumes, like beans)
- Nightshades: bell peppers (a.k.a. sweet peppers), eggplant, goji berries (a.k.a. wolfberry), hot peppers (such as chili peppers, jalapenos, habaneros, chili-based spices, red pepper, or cayenne), paprika, potatoes (but not sweet potatoes), tomatillos, and tomatoes
- Eggs
- Dairy
- Lentils
- Beans
- Quinoa
- Rice
- Other non-gluten grains
- Corn
- Sugar
- Gluten grains (wheat, rye, and barley): probably best to avoid altogether

I have a video posted on the "Workshops" page on my website called, "The Greatest Diet on the Planet" that goes through a step-by-step summary of how to follow the AI paleo diet. You can find it at www.innatechiro.

com/upcoming-workshops. And don't forget to check out autoimmunewellness.com. Angie and Mickey have a great site explaining the ins and outs of the AI paleo program. I recommend it to my patients as a reference all the time.

Every once in a while, whether it's once a year or every two years, you need to go through this process again. Once your body has set up a reaction to food or a food sensitivity, you can start reacting to different foods at different times—even to the things you were once okay with. Thus, it's important to do a reset every once in a while to see how you feel when you eat certain foods.

You can use the AI paleo diet as the baseline to determine which foods are good and which are bad for you. Once you know what foods your body uses as fuel—and doesn't react to—you're well on your way to improving your grade in food sensitivities and intolerances. You could create a whole new grade based on your adherence to the diet, your discipline in adding certain foods back in, and gradually getting the feedback from your body. Your adherence to the diet is very important, but remember, it's temporary. This is a tool to learn more about how your body reacts to foods. Overall, the thing to look for is steady improvement.

> **RULE:**
>
> If you think food sensitivities or food intolerances might be an issue for you, try the AI paleo program, and if you need further help, find a doctor to work with you.

> **RULE:**
>
> If your toxicity levels are high, reduce your exposure to external toxins. Increase the

detoxifying foods, supplements, and herbs you eat. Do a detox program that you trust every so often to reduce the toxic burden on your body.

IBS, Chronic Fatigue, and Frequent Colds: The 4R Program

If you are someone who deals with Irritable Bowel Syndrome, Chronic Fatigue, frequent colds, general malaise, or you just want to get healthier, then a 4R program may be right for you.

The 4R program is designed to be a digestive cleanse that resets the balance of flora in your gut for healthy digestion. There are many ways of cleansing, and through my experience, I have found that a doctor-prescribed, patient-tailored program achieves the best results. The four Rs stand for: Remove, Replace, Reinoculate, and Repair.

Gut flora are the living organisms (beneficial bacteria like acidophilus and bifidobacterium, yeasts, parasites, molds, and fungi) that reside in your intestinal tract. There are many colonies of these little microorganisms that live within us, and most are supposed to be there. If you knew how many microorganisms are living in and on your body, it would probably freak you out! There are actually more microorganisms living in and on your body than there are cells *in* your body. They outnumber us by a ratio of about ten to one. Our cells are much larger, though, so we take up much more space. A discussion on the ins and outs of our microbiome would require a multi-book series, so I'll simply default to having you Google "microbiome," if you are interested.

The beneficial or "good" bacteria and other microorganisms create a symbiotic relationship with your body. These microorganisms feast on your undigested food (mainly fiber), help your digestion, aid your immune system, and even assist you in producing helpful nutrients such as vitamin K.

Unfortunately, not all of the microorganisms that reside in your digestive tract are beneficial. Many strains of unfriendly microorganisms enter your body throughout your lifetime. These microorganisms don't help us—in fact, the *opposite* happens. These bad bugs can promote gas and toxins, which disturb the normal homeostasis of our bodies. The simple explanation I like to use in my office is this: "Good bugs live in our gut and help us by eating our poop and pooping out their own beneficial by-products. Bad bugs live in our gut and also eat our poop, but when they poop, they poop out toxins."

Dysbiosis is a term used to describe an imbalance of the gut flora. When the ratio of good to bad bugs gets out of control and the level of bad bacteria gets too high, we develop symptoms. That magic ratio is different for every individual, and the symptoms are quite varied. Symptoms can include chronic aches and pains, irregular bowel movements, loose stool, bloating, headaches, fatigue, and the list goes on. It's similar to the toxic symptoms mentioned previously.

The 4R Program

The 4R program has been used for many years in alternative medicine as a first line tool to help restore balance to the microbiome. I'll state it again: There is no substitute for getting advice from a medical/health professional before taking your health into your own hands. The purpose of all the information in this book is to help you understand different approaches that you or your current health practitioner may be unaware of so you can make the right choices when it comes to your healthcare.

The first R—*Removal*—addresses what to do with these bugs. The first step is to just get them out. There are many nutritional products available to help eliminate the bad microorganisms in your body. During the removal phase of the 4R Program, these supplements or medications are taken, and typically a yeast-free diet is recommended. Simply Google "yeast free diet" to understand what that means. This first phase of the process can last anywhere from two to eight weeks, depending on the individual. The goal of the diet is to remove the food/fuel so these "bad bugs" can't thrive.

The next R is *Replace.* Here, we replace digestive enzymes that help to ease the digestion of foods. At times, I also prescribe supplements that re-acidify the stomach with the proper betaine hydrochloride balance. The correct digestive enzymes will vary depending on the patient. This stage will be implemented along with one or more of the other Rs.

In the *Reinoculate* stage, beneficial bacteria and/or yeast supplements (probiotics) are prescribed to populate the digestive tract with high amounts of "good bugs." Again, the strains of probiotics that should be used are dependent on the individual. The length of time they're used and the dosages also vary.

I will state here that there is some confusing research pertaining to the use of probiotics. To sum it up, it seems that when you take probiotics, there is no definitive alteration in the makeup of the microorganism balance in the intestinal tract. On the other hand, the majority of studies state that there are favorable outcomes as far as symptoms are concerned.

I see two common problems in patients that are taking probiotics on their own. One is a lack of quality and stability. If a probiotic is dead by the time it reaches the target area, it is of no help. The second problem is a lack of knowledge regarding dosage (typically how many billions of probiotics to take per day) and how long they should be taken. I won't get into the specifics here because I believe in tailoring specific programs to the individual. This stage is usually more aggressive for four to eight weeks, then can last as long as six months or more. There are some people, myself included, who take probiotics on a regular basis because I usually find I feel better when taking them than when I'm not.

The last R is *Repair.* This stage involves testing for and adding in nutrients that will aid the digestive tract in its natural ability to repair itself. These nutrients can include turmeric, L-glutamine, B-vitamins, aloe, licorice and many others. Two of the most common products I use that are UltraInflam-X and Glutagenics by Metagenics and Repairvite by Apex Energetics. I do not mind mentioning these because of how many individuals I feel they have the potential to help. I reassess all the supplements I recommend from time to time, but these are common supplements I use now. This 'R' stage varies greatly in length. I have seen many individuals, including myself, use repair products such as UltraInflam-X for years, learning when to cycle on and off.

> **RULE:**
>
> If you're having IBS problems or are experiencing chronic fatigue or general malaise, find a health practitioner who can help guide you through a personalized 4R program.

Acid Reflux

Sometimes, I can't believe how many patients I see that have some form of acid reflux. It's hard to have straight As on your report card when acid reflux is showing up in the body. It's a clear indicator that something is off. If you have symptoms of reflux, here are some of the reasons *why* you might be getting them.

Symptoms can include upper abdominal bloating soon after a meal, a dry, persistent cough, persistently clearing your throat, bad breath, heartburn, or full-on burning acid regurgitating up to your mouth. There are many degrees of acid reflux, and all of them should be addressed. Letting small symptoms like these develop further could damage the esophagus and can even lead to cancers of the upper digestive tract.

The biggest problem I have with acid reflux is the most common approaches to treating it. Treating acid reflux usually means suppressing the acid with calcium (Tums) or various medications that inhibit the production of acid in the stomach. This approach may sound simple and may help you feel better, but there are consequences to suppressing or blocking acid. For one thing, our stomach is supposed to be a very acidic place. The acid from our stomach, mainly in the form of hydrochloric acid, helps us to digest our foods. Without the proper acidity levels, we have trouble digesting certain nutrients. Some of the more difficult to break down nutrients are minerals like calcium, magnesium, and many proteins (amino acids). Acid blocking can be necessary for short periods of time to allow the esophagus to heal, but staying on these acid reducers can lead to other problems stemming from the loss of these vital nutrients.

Of course, I cannot mention acid reflux without first recommending that if you feel that you have any medical condition, seek the advice of a medical doctor—in this case, a gastroenterologist. I hope I have made the point clear enough in this book that my philosophy is to treat the *person with the symptom, not the symptom itself.* I do see many people with heartburn or acid reflux or many other symptoms that *I don't treat!* I address all symptoms with the same approach ... find out which physical, chemical, and emotional stresses or imbalances the person is dealing with, and help them to be healthier! I have found great success over the past two decades by simply doing this. When the approach I'm taking isn't getting results, I always get a second or even a third opinion by referring to another health practitioner who specializes in dealing with that symptom.

My approach to helping people who have symptoms of acid reflux is to address the deficiencies or structural imbalances that led to the symptoms in the first place. That is always the treatment approach at our office—treat the person, not the symptom. Some of the common issues that we see in our office when someone has acid reflux are either a zinc deficiency, a B12 deficiency, a hiatal hernia, a TMJ (jaw) problem, a poor diet, or a subluxation (misalignment) of the mid-cervical or thoracic vertebrae. Usually, it is a combination of a few or all of these problems. Of course, there are other causes as well.

As an example, I will begin by explaining a very common pattern I find in my office: the relationship of a TMJ imbalance and people with acid reflux. It starts off with the trigger for every problem—*stress*. No matter what kind of stress they're experiencing, one of the things people do when under stress is to clench their teeth together, placing stress on the temporomandibular joint (TMJ) or jaw joint. Sometimes, people are only doing this at night while asleep, and if it weren't for their partner or their dentist, they wouldn't even be aware of it. If there happens to be even a slight imbalance in the alignment of your bite, then that clenching or grinding of your teeth can cause TMJ discomfort or dysfunction. As soon as the innate intelligence of our body senses TMJ dysfunction, there should be a compensation to alleviate that dysfunction.

Your jaw is very important! If it doesn't work properly, you don't eat, and you die. So preserving the function of the jaw takes priority over many other problems. The classic compensation I find for a jaw problem is to create tension in muscles around the neck area to help bring the jaw back into alignment. If that muscular compensation subluxates (misaligns) the third, fourth, or fifth cervical bones, there can be an impact on the function of your diaphragm (C3, C4, C5—all innervate the diaphragm muscle), and a weakness in the diaphragm muscle can lead to a hiatal hernia.

A hiatal hernia happens when a weakness in the diaphragm allows a part of the stomach to rise up above the diaphragm where the esophagus should be. Why is that a problem? There is a small sphincter that separates the esophagus and the stomach. That sphincter keeps the acid in the stomach. In the case of the hiatal hernia, that sphincter may not be working properly, and acid or regurgitated food can escape. When there is a problem with the optimum function of the diaphragm, there can be tension that builds up in the fifth, sixth, and/or seventh thoracic vertebrae, which all contribute to the innervation (nerve supply) of the stomach itself.

When there is a zinc or B-12 deficiency or insufficiency, there may be a decrease in the production of hydrochloric acid in the stomach. Insufficient hydrochloric acid can also lead to acid reflux. Sounds crazy, I know—not enough acid causing acid reflux? But if there is enough acid in the stomach, that acidity actually helps that sphincter we mentioned at the junction of the stomach and the diaphragm to close. With a lack of acidity, that sphincter can get "lazy," and if there is too little acid to stimulate it to close, it can become weak. If you have a weak sphincter and you eat a meal that will temporarily increase your stomach acidity, that acid can escape out of the weakened valve and give you symptoms of acid reflux. If you have the proper acidity, your acid reflux can improve.

The way to fix all of this is to see a healthcare practitioner who understands all of these working parts. This is why I love applied kinesiology so much; it gives the practitioner the tools to understand why the patient is having symptoms from many different perspectives, without the use of drugs or surgery.

The typical protocol in our office involves checking for and fixing subluxations in the spine and the TMJ by adjusting and/or using muscle balancing techniques. Also, we check for dietary and supplemental betaine hydrochloride, digestive enzymes, zinc, and B vitamins. We can also release stress from the diaphragm itself with different muscular corrections. This, of course, is one of the many common patterns I see in *patients who have* reflux. In the end, every person I see has slightly different stresses, and our goal is to work through them individually, piece by piece.

The longer you have had these imbalances, the more difficult they are to fix, but given time, most people can get healthy without the use of drugs or surgery.

> **RULE:**
> If you're having any symptom, find a health practitioner who will help you find the *cause* rather than simply treating the symptom.

Chronic Pain

If you're having chronic pain, it's important to first understand that pain itself is not a *problem*; pain is a *symptom.* That may be a difficult "pill to swallow" for someone currently in pain, but it's true.

Let's say you have chronic headaches. How I would address a patient with chronic headaches would be to first examine them to figure out what type of physical stress they are carrying in their neck. If there are subluxations (misalignments of the spine leading to stress on the nervous system) and soft tissue imbalances (knots in the muscle or fascia) then those may actually be a primary source of the pain experienced in your head.

Next, I would ask them about their lifestyle, including work, exercise habits, diet, sleep habits ... all of the key points in the report card. There may be two, three, or even more separate lifestyle issues that, if they were addressed, would solve the cause of their headaches.

If we can understand that pain is not a problem but, rather, a *signal* of a problem, we can go to work fixing the source of the problem. Pain is actually our friend. It can tell us when we're out of alignment and can signal to us that we need to make changes.

More about Stress and Tension Headaches

It's possible that you're having issues with chronic headaches. One estimate states that almost half of all adults all over the world have had a headache within the last year.[6] It's been found up to 43 percent of the reported headaches are tension-type headaches.[7] While migraines tend to be chemical-based and tension-type headaches can be emotionally based, a lot of headaches are caused by structural/physical problems.

I have found over the past twenty years of practice that many headaches are cervicogenic headaches, meaning that the cause of the headache comes from abnormalities in the muscles, joints, or fascia of the neck. The major thing that most people don't pay attention to when it comes to the neck is its curvature. Our heads are supposed to be sitting on a nice, flexible curve in the neck called a lordosis. When there is a loss of the cervical lordosis, it creates tension in the soft tissue of the neck that can ultimately lead to many types of pain, including headaches. When you have a loss of the normal cervical lordosis—or even worse, a reversal of the normal curve so that it's now kyphotic, or curved in the opposite direction—your spine will suffer from an increased rate of degeneration.[8] Your discs wear down, and the muscles around your neck area become tense.

Remember: this is only one reason for pain! I have consistently found that the main reason someone "feels" the pain of these degenerative changes is because they are also dealing with an accumulation of other physical, chemical, or emotional stress. The loss of lordosis in the neck will cause degenerative changes that you may or may not feel on a regular basis, so it's best to be evaluated by a trained doctor of chiropractic to determine how it is affecting your overall health."

Also, one specific type of headache can develop if the muscles right at the second cervical—just below the base of your skull on either side—tense up. This can affect something called your *greater occipital nerve*, which is a nerve that runs from the back of your neck up to the back of your head. This type of headache can radiate pain to the area around the eye. I have found that many headaches that wrap around to the eye area are relieved by addressing the subluxations and soft tissue imbalances in this area through chiropractic care.

If you're having tension headaches regularly, I would recommend seeing a chiropractor to work on your alignment (refer to the chapter on *Alignment*). What do most of us do about our headaches? Pop a pill! You're not experiencing a headache because of a lack of acetaminophen or ibuprofen in your life... . I would suggest, as with any symptom you feel, that you always try to figure out the cause rather than just temporarily alleviate your pain. I want you to think about any chronic pain, as mild or as severe as it may be, in a similar way. I want you to ask yourself—and ask your doctor—*why* the pain is there is the first place. If you don't know the answer, find someone who will help you. But don't wait! Start improving your HPA, and your pain will most likely get better.

> **RULE:**
>
> If you're having chronic pain or headaches, the first doctor to visit is a chiropractor.

> **Overall RULE for Special Circumstances:**
>
> Track your progress on your custom grading scale for any special circumstances you're experiencing in your health and quality of life. Work toward regular improvement!

Keep the Momentum

Congratulations! You've gone through the entire book on how to raise your grades in each of the areas of life on your Personal Report Card (PRC). As a summary, this tool provides you with three main things: (1) the ability to know where you're at right now, (2) the ability to know how to get better, and (3) the ability to know if what you're doing between report cards is working.

Remember that the title of this book is *Better*. It's not called *Perfect* or *The Best*. The report card is about making improvements that will elevate your quality of life, now and for the rest of your life.

How can you know if you're getting better? By completing the report card more than once. Your PRC is a *continual process*. To get the most out of what you've learned in this book, keep filling out report cards repeatedly throughout the year and compare your grades. Filling it out once will tell you where you're at right now, but it won't use the power of the tool to its fullest; you won't know how much you've improved from one time to the next, if at all.

To apply this tool successfully, you'll have to build up some momentum. Schedule the times on your calendar throughout the year when you're going to fill out a new

PRC. As mentioned previously, my recommendation is to fill one out every quarter or every solstice. Spring, summer, fall, winter. . . they should all be a trigger for you to fill out a new report card and calculate your Health Point Average (HPA).

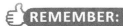

REMEMBER:

There is a tool on my website to help you calculate your HPA at www.innatechiro.com.

RULE:

Designate and schedule times to fill out your report card again and again throughout the year. To gain momentum, stick to this schedule and adjust your grading scales as frequently as needed in order to keep yourself moving forward in all areas. Try a quarterly/seasonal report card.

If you feel yourself slipping or losing momentum, revisit the area of the book where you're stuck. Go back to the *Habits* section at the beginning of the book. Refresh your memory on how to anchor new habits and follow through with them. Use this book as a resource as you go from one report to the next. You may need to read the whole book several times; that's okay—I wrote this book as a long-term partner and support structure for you to continually improve your life and your health.

As we talked about in this book, progress is not always seamless, steady, or universal. You might not be seeing much progress in one area, but that's because your body needs to focus on improving in another area first. For example, you might not notice drastic improvements in the area of *Sleep* until you improve your grades in *Exercise* and *Supplements*. This doesn't mean your sleep isn't going to improve—it means your body requires you to make other changes *in conjunction with* instilling new sleep habits to see big improvement. This will take time.

Sometimes, improvements happen quickly in one area, sometimes you can see gradual improvements in a couple of areas, and at other times, you might not see any improvements at all from one report card to another—in one area or maybe even in all of them. This doesn't mean failure; it simply means it's time to reassess your rules, habits, and grading scales.

If you find yourself feeling overwhelmed, or you feel like the results you're striving for are over your head, it will be more challenging to stay in the game. But here's the secret: Reassessing your grading scales, outgrowing them, and needing to adjust them is *part* of the game—one of the most important parts. You will gain momentum by thinking of your report card as a dynamic extension of yourself. This means you can change your report card based upon your changing needs. Doing so will keep you connected to your goals, progress, and the habits that are taking you to new levels.

Even the best version of yourself is dynamic. That means there is no final destination when you are focused on getting *better*; there is no moment when you say, "Okay, I've arrived," and that's it. If you focus on being *better*, rather than reaching a static version of what you consider *the best*, you'll find that you will always move forward because *you can always be better.*

The key to progress is participation. Stay in the game and *keep going.* Focus on the areas where you feel great and where you are seeing improvements. Celebrate your successes. Keep up your habits, even in areas where you aren't seeing much initial improvement.

And, most importantly, remember to have fun with your report card! Allow yourself to enjoy the process. Push yourself to grow, but don't be too hard on yourself. Remember that your mindset and how you feel along the way are essential to improvement. Make sure you're taking care of yourself while you're pushing yourself to grow and keep up with new habits. If you fall off, don't judge yourself—just get back on! Don't expect perfection. Use the section on *Connectedness* and *Stress Management* to help you stay positive.

If you need extra support, visit my website at **www.innatechiro.com**. There, you will have access to workshops and videos that will provide even more information and tips to help you continue improving.

This is just the beginning to a better you; I am so glad that you're on your way. Onwards and upwards!

> **RULE:**
>
> Keep going! Listen to the feedback your body gives you, adjust your habits and rules accordingly, and stay the course.

Appendix

RULE: Make your own rules that work for *you*.

RULE: Anchor your rules to daily tasks so you remember to do them!

RULE: Add one new good food or positive habit into your life every few weeks until your grade is better.

RULE: Stop. Take out things that are not serving you anymore.

RULE: Don't *try* anything. If you want something to change, make a *decision* to change it *now*! Set a time limit for how long you will carry out the change. Don't make any promises to yourself that you can't keep!

RULE: Wake up early and get out of the house!

RULE: Eat breakfast within the first hour of waking up! Start your day with food, not junk.

RULE: Set the tone for your day. Create and implement a morning routine that sets you in a powerful, positive direction!

RULE: Listen to your innate intelligence about any symptoms you're having and look for the solution in changing your food rules and habits.

RULE: Eat frequently—at least four times a day!

RULE: For lunch, *just have a freakin' salad*!

RULE: Don't have dinner be your biggest meal of the day. Find out what foods are best for *your* body and eat those foods in a portion comparable to your other meals of the day.

RULE: Just stop eating junk food! And if you still find yourself tempted, create a rule that limits how much of it you eat.

RULE: Overall, when it comes to food, conventional is necessary, organic is better, and wild is best.

RULE: Take supplements. We may not need them to survive, but we do need them to *thrive*. If you want to get the most out of life, just take them.

RULE: Learn what supplements are right for you. Consult a healthcare professional for guidance or hit the books and start learning.

RULE: *Exercise*! It is not an option! In some way, shape, or form, on a very regular basis, you *must* Exercise if you want to be healthy!

RULE: Get moving! Use the ratio of time/intensity. Learn how to exercise better.

RULE: If it will take you more than six weeks to have the body of your dreams, then get to work!

RULE: Only buy workout equipment and services you will actually *use*.

RULE: Exercise makes you *smile*! You're only one workout away from a good mood!

RULE: Throw away your scale and work on your shape!

RULE: Sleep = healing. Sleep six to nine hours a night.

RULE: Use proper pillow techniques and switch sides of the bed often. The pillow I recommend most these days? **Mypillow.com**

RULE: Sleep is a time to rest, repair, and heal. If you're having trouble sleeping, improve your grades in all areas of your life and create and follow a nighttime ritual. If you're still having trouble sleeping, get to a sleep clinic to improve your quality of sleep.

RULE: Drink half your body weight in fluid ounces of water a day. If you're still thirsty on top of that because of a hot day or a hard workout, drink extra water to quench your thirst or add in coconut water. To avoid constant bathroom breaks, set up the optimal times throughout your day to drink water.

RULE: Kick off your shoes once a day and roll your feet over a tennis ball.

RULE: Take breaks throughout your work day. Keep your body moving. Eat lunch away from your desk!

RULE: Implement one new stress-reducing strategy each year and prioritize it.

RULE: Reconnect with yourself. Spend at least twenty-four hours with *just you.*

RULE: If you haven't been practicing meditation, begin as soon as possible!

RULE: *Only* speak about yourself in a positive manner. Even in jest, your words are powerful—especially what you say about yourself!

RULE: When you feel your mind is racing and you simply cannot sit and close your eyes and meditate, try a twenty-minute walk where you are mindful of your surroundings and your breath and nothing else!

RULE: Follow @Drpiken on Twitter and "like" Innate Chiropractic of Manhattan on Facebook—I only post articles, audios, and videos that will increase your grade in *Health Awareness*!

RULE: To stay regular and have a healthy elimination process, follow the four rules for healthy elimination: fiber, water, microorganisms, and magnesium.

RULE: If you think food sensitivities or food intolerances might be an issue for you, try the AI paleo

program, and if you need further help, find a
doctor to work with you.

RULE: If your toxicity levels are high, reduce your
exposure to external toxins. Increase the
detoxifying foods, supplements, and herbs you
eat. Do a detox program that you trust every so
often to reduce the toxic burden on your body.

RULE: If you're having IBS problems or are experiencing
chronic fatigue or general malaise, find a health
practitioner who can help guide you through a
personalized 4R program.

RULE: If you're having any symptom, find a health
practitioner who will help you find the *cause*
rather than simply treating the symptom.

RULE: If you're having chronic pain or headaches, the
first doctor to visit is a chiropractor.

Overall RULE for Special Circumstances: Track your
progress on your custom grading scale for any
special circumstances you're experiencing in your
health and quality of life. Work toward regular
improvement!

RULE: Designate and schedule times to fill out your
report card again and again throughout the year.
To gain momentum, stick to this schedule and
adjust your grading scales as frequently as needed
in order to keep yourself moving forward in all
areas. Try a quarterly/seasonal report card.

RULE: Keep going! Listen to the feedback your body gives you, adjust your habits and rules accordingly, and stay the course!

BMI	19	20	21	22	23	24	25	26	27	28	29	30	31	32	33	34	35
HEIGHT in inches							Body weight in pounds										
58	91	96	100	105	110	115	119	124	129	134	138	143	148	153	158	162	167
59	94	99	104	109	114	119	124	128	133	138	143	148	153	158	163	168	173
60	97	102	107	112	118	123	128	133	138	143	148	153	158	163	168	174	179
61	100	106	111	116	122	127	132	137	143	148	153	158	164	169	174	180	185
62	104	109	115	120	126	131	136	142	147	153	158	164	169	175	180	186	191
63	107	113	118	124	130	135	141	146	152	158	163	169	175	180	186	191	197
64	110	116	122	128	134	140	145	151	157	163	169	174	180	186	192	197	204
65	114	120	126	132	138	144	150	156	162	168	174	180	186	192	198	204	210
66	118	124	130	136	142	148	155	161	167	173	179	186	192	198	204	210	216
67	121	127	134	140	146	153	159	166	172	178	185	191	198	204	211	217	223
68	125	131	138	144	151	158	164	171	177	184	190	197	203	210	216	223	230
68	128	135	142	149	155	162	169	176	182	189	196	203	209	216	223	230	236
70	132	139	146	153	160	167	174	181	188	195	202	209	216	222	229	236	243
71	136	143	150	157	165	172	179	186	193	200	208	215	222	229	236	243	250
72	140	147	154	162	169	177	184	191	199	206	213	221	228	235	242	250	258
73	144	151	159	166	174	182	189	197	204	212	219	227	235	242	250	257	265
74	148	155	163	171	179	186	194	202	210	218	225	233	241	249	256	264	272
75	152	160	168	176	184	192	200	208	216	224	232	240	248	256	264	272	279
76	156	164	172	180	189	197	205	213	221	230	238	246	254	263	271	279	287

Piken
Recommends

List of books to read for more info, based on what Dr. Piken has read.

1. *Chicken Soup for the Soul* by Jack Canfield and Mark Victor Hansen
2. *No More Allergies* by Gary Null
3. *Total Renewal* by Frank Lipman, MD
4. *The Road Less Traveled* by M. Scott Peck, MD
5. *Eat, Drink, and Be Healthy* by Walter C. Willett, MD
6. *Kabbalah for the Layman, Volume 1* by Rabbi Berg
7. *10% Happier* by Dan Harris
8. *The Teachings of Don Juan* by Carlos Castaneda
9. *Sorcerer's Apprentice* by Carlos Castaneda
10. *The Art of Dreaming* by Carlos Castaneda
11. *Awaken the Giant Within* by Anthony Robbins
12. *The Power of Intention* by Wayne Dyer
13. *Excuses Begone!* by Wayne Dyer
14. *Living the Wisdom of the Tao* by Wayne Dyer
15. *Change Your Thoughts, Change Your Life* by Wayne Dyer
16. *10 Secrets of Success and Inner Peace* by Wayne Dyer
17. *The Power of Now* by Eckhart Tolle

18. *The Way* by Michael Berg
19. *Oh, the Places You'll Go* by Dr. Seuss
20. *My Stroke of Insight* by Jill Bolt Taylor, PhD
21. *The Hidden Brain* by Shankar Vedantam
22. *Why Isn't My Brain Working?* by Datis Kharrazian DHSc, DC, MS
23. *Why Do I Still Have Thyroid Symptoms?* by Datis Kharrazian DHSc, DC, MS
24. *A People's History of the United States* by Howard Zinn
25. *Don't Know Much about History* by Kenneth C. Davis
26. *Drunk Tank Pink* by Adam Alter
27. *The Holographic Universe* by Michael Talbot
28. *The Power of Positive Thinking* by Norman Vincent Peale
29. *Power vs. Force* by David R. Hawkins
30. *The Tao of Pooh* by Benjamin Hoff
31. *The I Ching* by Lao Tsu
32. *The Tao of Inner Peace* by Diane Dreher
33. *Conversations with God* by Neale Donald Walsh
34. *Happier* by Tal Ben-Shahar
35. *How to Raise a Healthy Child in Spite of Your Doctor* by Robert S. Mendelsohn, MD
36. *Crazy Sexy Diet* by Kris Carr
37. *The Power of Myth* by Joseph Campbell
38. *The Four Agreements* by Don Miguel Ruiz
39. *The Monk Who Sold His Ferrari* by Robin S. Sharma
40. *The 17 Essential Qualities of a Team Player* by John C. Maxwell
41. *Waking the Tiger* by Ann Frederick and Peter A Levine

42. *Influencer* by Al Switzler, David Maxfield, Joseph Grenny, and Kerry Patterson
43. *Walking the Walk* by Leslie Sansone
44. *Getting Unstuck* by Pema Chodron
45. *Ego is the Enemy* by Ryan Holiday
46. *The Happiness Advantage* by Shawn Achor
47. *The E Myth* by Michael E. Gerber
48. *Brain Maker* by Kristin Loberg and David Perlmutter, MD
49. *Clarity* by Jamie Smart
50. *Blink* by Malcolm Gladwell

@drpiken

www.facebook.com/innatechiromanhattan/

W ebsite recommendations:

www.innatechiro.com
brianjohnson.me
Seancroxton.com
Undergroundwellness.com
Autoimmunewellness.com
thedr.com
mindvalleyacademy.com
audiodharma.org
pemachodronfoundation.org
www.ted.com

References

Calbourne, Cherie. *The Juice Lady's Remedies for Stress and Adrenal Fatigue.* Siloam. www.charismahouse.com

Centers for Disease Control and Prevention. "Insufficient Sleep is a Public Health Problem" https://www.cdc.gov/features/dssleep/ (online). Retrieved November 6, 2016.

Francis, Raymond. *Never Be Sick Again.* Health Communications Inc. Deerfield Beach, Florida.

Hoffman, Bob and Jason Deitch. *Discover Wellness: How Staying Healthy Can Make You Rich.* Center Path Publishing

Hong-Mei Zhang, Lei Zhao, Hao Li, Hao Xu, Wen-Wen Chen and Lin Tao. "Research Progress on the Anticarcinogenic Actions and Mechanisms of Ellagic Acid. *Cancer Biol Med.* Jun 2014. 11(2): 92–100.

Hyman, Mark, MD, and Mark Liponis, MD. *Ultraprevention.* Atria Books.

Junger, Alejandro, MD. *Clean.* HarperCollins.com.

Pari L, and Satheesh MA. "Effect of Pterostilbene on Hepatic Key Enzymes of Glucose Metabolism in Streptozotocin- and Nicotinamide-Induced Diabetic Rats." *Life Sciences.* 2006 Jul 10;79(7):641-5.

Phillips, Bill. *Body for Life.* Harper Collins

Pollan, Michael. *Food Rules.* Penguin Books.

Rimando AM, Nagmani R, Feller DR and Yokoyama W. "Pterostilbene, a New Agonist for the Peroxisome Proliferator-Activated Receptor Alpha-Isoform,

Lowers Plasma Lipoproteins and Cholesterol in Hypercholesterolemic Hamsters." *Journal of Agriculture and Food Chemistry*. 2005 May 4;53(9):3403-7.

Rozen, Michael, MD and Mehmet Oz, MD. *You: The Owner's Manual*. Harper Collins.

Tarcher, Jeremy P., PhD and Mark Mincolla. *Whole Health*. Penguin Books.

Xia Jinghe, Toshihiko Mizuta, and Iwata Ozaki. "Vitamin K and Hepatocellular Carcinoma: The Basic and Clinic." *World Journal of Clinical Cases*. 2015 Sep 16; 3(9): 757–764.

Notes

1. A Values taken from: Kyle UG, et al. "Fat-Free and Fat Mass Percentiles in 5225 Healthy Subjects Aged 15 to 98 Years." Nutrition, 17:534–541, 2001.

2. Whitney, Paul, PhD and John M. Hinson, PhD and Melinda L. Jackson, PhD and Hans P.A. Van Dongen, PhD. "Feedback Blunting: Total Sleep Deprivation Impairs Decision Making that Requires Updating Based on Feedback." *Sleep.* 2015 May 1; 38(5): 745–754. Published online 2015 May 1. doi: 10.5665/sleep.4668. PMCID: PMC4402662. https://www.ncbi.nlm.nih.gov/pmc/articles/PMC4402662/ Nov 6.

3. Mah, Cheri D., MS, and Kenneth E. Mah, MD, MS and Eric J. Kezirian, MD, MPH and William C. Dement, MD, PhD. "The Effects of Sleep Extension on the Athletic Performance of Collegiate Basketball Players." *Sleep.* 2011 Jul 1; 34(7): 943–950. Published online 2011 Jul 1. doi: 10.5665/SLEEP.1132. PMCID: PMC3119836. https://www.ncbi.nlm.nih.gov/pmc/articles/PMC3119836/ Nov 6.

4. Jackson, Melinda L. and Glenn Gunzelmann and Paul Whitney and John M. Hinson and Gregory Belenky and Arnaud Rabat and Hans P. A. Van Dongena. "Deconstructing and Reconstructing Cognitive Performance in Sleep Deprivation." *Sleep* Med Rev. Author manuscript; available in PMC 2014 Jun 1. Published in final edited form as: *Sleep* Med Rev. 2013 Jun; 17(3): 215–225. Published online 2012 Aug 9. doi: 10.1016/j.smrv.2012.06.007.

PMCID: PMC3498579. NIHMSID: NIHMS392242. https://www.ncbi.nlm.nih.gov/pmc/articles/PMC3498579/ Nov 6.

5. Adv Nutr March 2011 Adv Nutr vol. 2: 151-152, 2011.

6. http://www.who.int/mediacentre/factsheets/fs277/en/

7. https://www.ncbi.nlm.nih.gov/pubmed/17381554

8. Eur, Spine J. "The association between cervical spine curvature and neck pain." 2007 May; 16(5): 669–678. Published online 2006 Nov 18. doi: 10.1007/s00586-006-0254-1. PMCID: PMC2213543.

About the Author

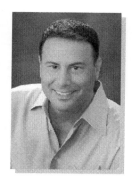

Dr. Jason Piken is the owner of Innate Chiropractic of Manhattan. A 1996 graduate of New York Chiropractic College, he became proficient in Gonstead, a system of analyzing the spine, and has since spent hundreds of seminar-hours broadening his technique skills to include Chiropractic Biophysics and Applied Kinesiology.

Dr. Piken is also a Certified Nutrition Specialist. He is an avid reader and is constantly engaged in learning to improve his understanding of nutrition and how to better care for the physical, chemical, and emotional well-being of the thousands of people he has had the honor of serving. Dr. Piken is a member of the New York Chiropractic Council and the American College of Nutrition and participates in many volunteer community outreach programs.

Growing up in Queens, New York, Dr. Piken knew all his life that the best of everything was found in NYC! That is why he chose to practice in the heart of New York City. If you want to provide the best healthcare, setting up where the best of everything is located only makes sense.

With a heavy focus on nutrition and a total-body approach to your health, Dr. Piken's office functions as a primary source for healthcare without the use of drugs or surgery. Applied Kinesiology and functional laboratory analysis are key systems used at Innate Chiropractic to expertly address the three basic causes of all health problems: chemical, emotional, and structural.

Dr. Piken lives in Westchester, NY with his wife, two children, and two rescued dogs.

Made in the USA
Middletown, DE
04 February 2017